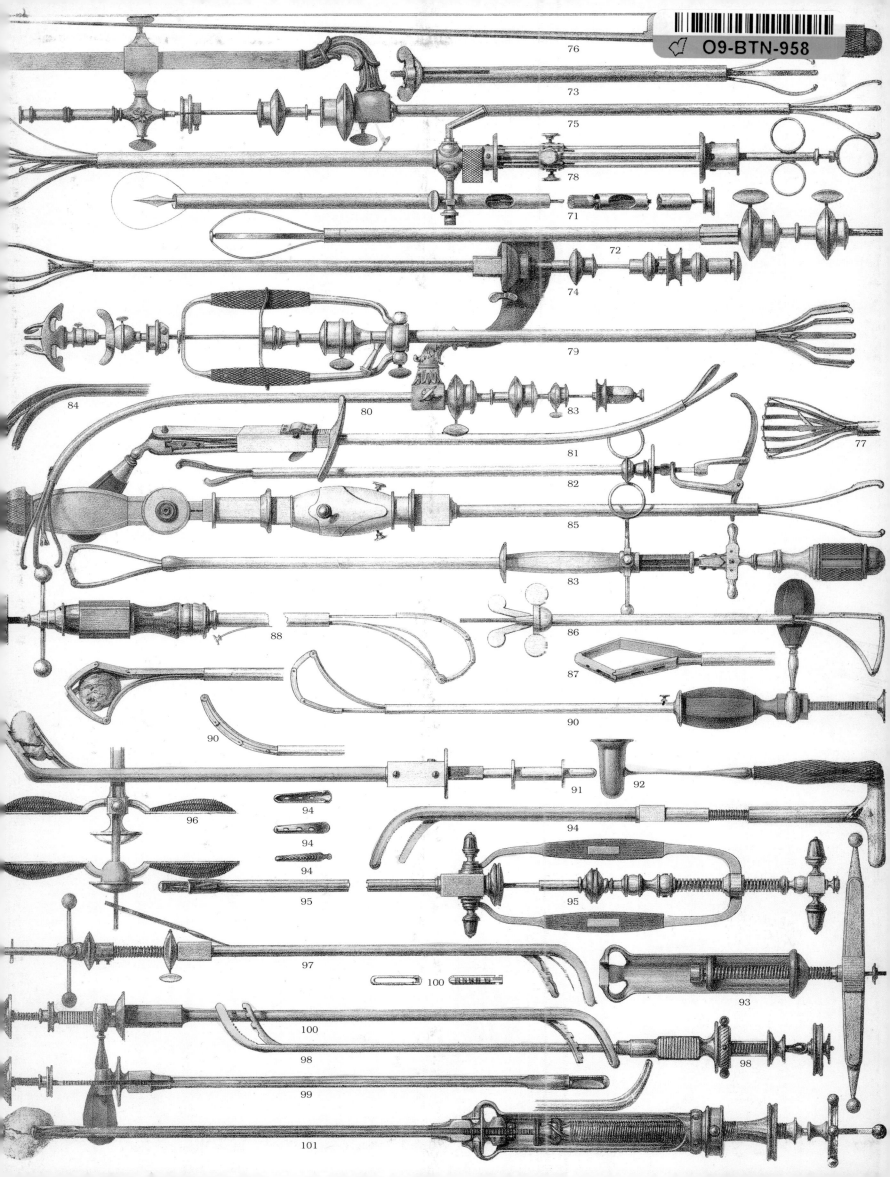

**Key to instruments on front end paper**

## Surgical instruments used in or via the urethra

**1° Catherisation**

Figures 1-9:
Silver catheters, with varying curves and volumes, for catherisation in men

Figure 10:
Catheter used to look for calculus in the bladder

Figure 11:
Straight catheters

Figure 12:
Acoustic tube. The tip is inserted into a catheter, and the ivory horn applied to the ear

Figures 13:
Conical catheter, used for forced catherisation

Figure 14:
Dual flow catheter, used for bladder irrigations

**2° Stenosis of the urethra**

Figures 15, 27-28:
Explanatory instruments

Figures 16-23:
Dilators

Figures 23, 24:
Depressors for hypertrophied prostrate.

Figures 29-35:
Cauterising instruments

Figures 36-48:
Scarificators used to puncture the skin

**3° Urethral lithotripsy**

Figures 49-64:
Instruments used to break down or extract calculus in the bladder

**4° Ligature of the prostrate** (median lobe, pathological)

Figures 65-66:
Cannulas

**5° Vices to fix the lithotripsy instruments for the bladder**

These are shown in figures 67-70

## Lithotripsy instruments for the bladder

**Instruments which work by progressive wearing away followed by pulverisation**

Figures 71-80:
Eccentric abrasion or perforation

Figures 81-84:
Concentric or peripheral abrasion

**Instruments which simply crush the calculus by gradual and continual pressure**

These are shown in figures 85-90

**Crushing or pulverisation instruments which work by simple or gradual pressure or by percussion**

These are shown in figures 91-101

# TIMETABLES OF MEDICINE

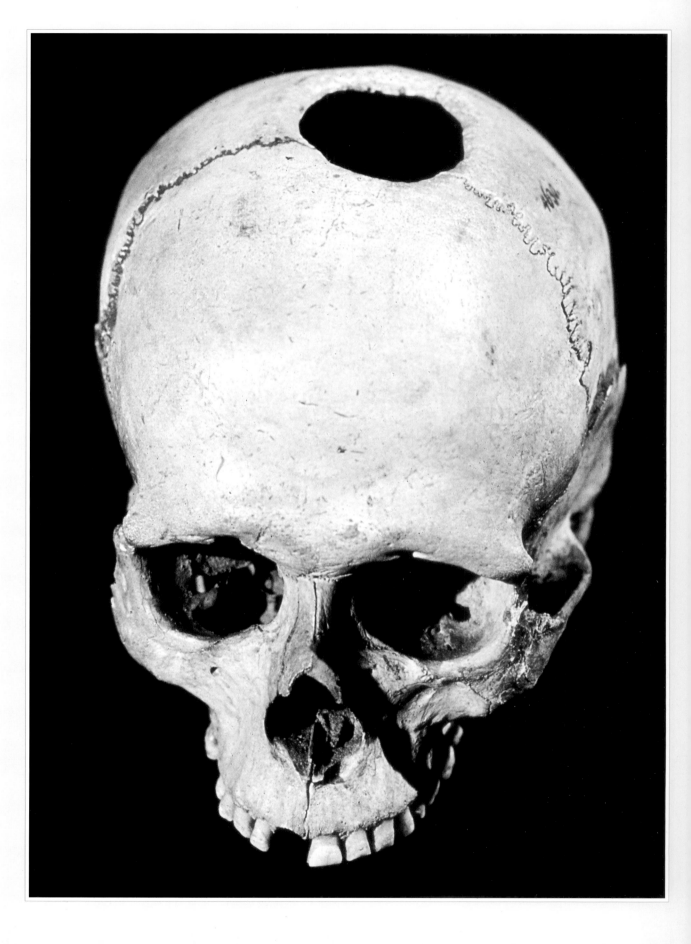

**Prehistory**
*Trephined skulls are the first evidence of surgery. Smooth healed bone edges indicate that some, at least, of the victims survived their ordeal, and multiple holes that repeated operations were not unknown*

**20th Century**
*An MRI (Magnetic Resonance Imaging) scan of a human head: the new technologies, including scanning and computer controlled lasers, enable precise and non-invasive surgery*

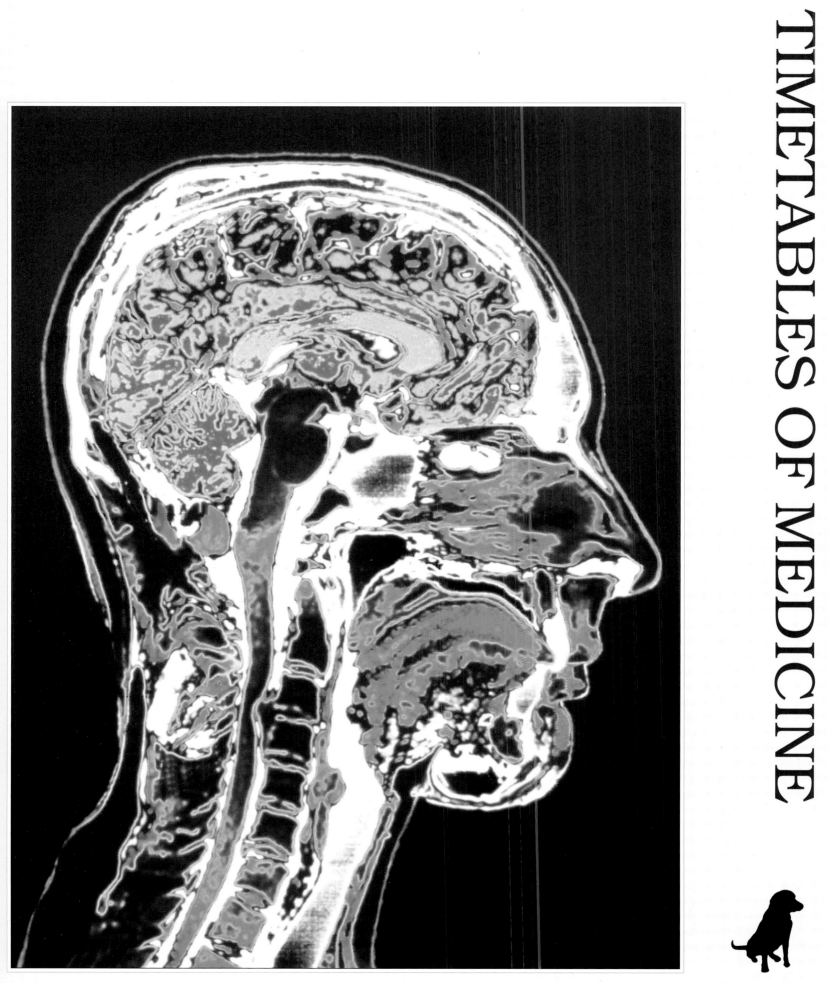

TIMETABLES OF MEDICINE

BLACK DOG
& LEVENTHAL
PUBLISHERS

This edition published by
**Black Dog & Leventhal**,
by arrangement with
Worth Press Limited.

© Worth Press Limited 2000

First published 1999 by
**The Timechart Company**
an imprint of
Worth Press Limited
9 Batchworth Heath
Rickmansworth
Hertfordshire
WD3 1QB

Published by
Black Dog & Leventhal
Publishers
151 West 19th Street
New York NY 10011

Distributed by
Workman Publishing
Company
708 Broadway
New York NY 10003

ISBN 1-57912-156-X

CIP catalogue records for
this book are available from
the British Library and the
Library of Congress.

**Timetables of Medicine**
was conceived, edited
and designed by
**Playne Books Limited**
Chapel House
Trefin, Haverfordwest
Pembrokeshire SA62 5AU
United Kingdom

*Compiled and edited by*
**Gill Davies**

*Consultant editor*
**Dr John Cule**

*Consultant*
**Professor Roy Porter**

*Editorial and research*
Janice Douglas

*Designers and illustrators*
Jonathan Douglas
David Playne

*Picture research*
Gill Playne
Kathryn Kelly

*French translation*
Michelle Evans

*Typeset by*
Playne Books Limited
in Bookman

Printed in China

*The publishers wish to thank:*

**Professor Roy Porter**
MA PhD (cantab) FBA
HonFRCP for writing the
*Introduction* and for his
advice and help.

Roy Porter is Professor in the
Social History of Medicine at
the Wellcome Institute for
the History of Medicine in
London. He has taught at the
University of Cambridge and
at UCLA in the USA.
Professor Roy Porter has
written and edited many
influential books.

**Doctor John Cule**
MD FRCGP FSA for his help
in the checking of data and
considerable advice about
the compilation of this book.

Doctor John Cule is Head
of the Medical History Unit,
University of Wales College
of Medicine. He has practised
clinical medicine both as a
family general practitioner
and also as a hospital
psychiatrist. He is currently
joint editor of *Vesalius*, the
journal of the International
Society for the History of
Medicine and has been
involved in many societies
over the years.

His appointments include
President of the International
Society for the History
of Medicine, President of
the British Society for the
History of Medicine and
President of the History of
Medicine Society of Wales.
Made an Emeritus Member
of the American Osler Society
in 1990 and elected an
Honorary Fellow of the Royal
Society of Medicine in 1996,
John Cule is also the author,
contributor to, and editor
of many books.

*Special thanks to:*

**Dr Peter G Skew** for further
advice. Dr Skew has been in
General Practice in the
private sector for fifteen
years. He specialises in
musculoskeletal medicine
and is Vice President of the
British Institute of
Musculoskeletal Medicine.
He has recently been elected
to the Executive Committee
of the Board of Trustees of
the National Back Pain
Association.

**Dr Lesley Hall** The UK
milestones described in
the section on *Women* were
largely drawn from
information compiled by
Dr Lesley Hall, to whom we
are very grateful.

**Medical Women's
Federation**, London.

**OrthoPrep Limited,**
Gloucestershire.

**David R S Pearson**
Librarian at The Wellcome
Institute for the History
of Medicine.

**The Wellcome Institute
Library** London, and the
individual librarians who
gave so much help.

*The Publishers wish to thank the following
for the use of pictures and photographs*

AKG, London 2, 5, 11, 22-23, 24-25, 26-27, 32-33
Amsterdam Historisch Museum, Netherlands 30-31
Antiquarium in the Residez, Munich 22-23
Archaeological Museum, Ankara, Turkey 20-21
Ashwell Editions 5, 34-35, 36
Bibliotheque Nationale, Paris 20-21, 24-25
Bibliotheque Royale Albert, Brussels 24-25
Bodleian Library, Oxford 24-25
Bridgeman Art Library/Lauros-Giraudon 20-21, 22-23
The British Library, London 13, 24-25
British Museum 20-21
British School of Osteopathy 18
Collection Putti Instituto Rizzoli, Bologna, 24-25
Collection William Helfand, New York 30-31, 32-33
Colorific 36
Corbis-Bettman 11, 34-35
Dr Jeremy Burgess 26-27
Egyptian Museum, Cairo 20-21
E.T. Archive 5, 8, 14, 15, 22-23, 26-27, 32-33
Fratelli Fabbri, Mila, 24-25
Gemälde-Galerie, Berlin 24-25
Indian Museum, Calcutta 20-21
Jefferson Medical College, Philadelphia, USA 7
Kupferstichkabinett Staatlich Museen
    Preussischer Kulturbisitz, Berlin, 26-27
Library of Congress, Washington D.C. USA 12
London College of Physicians 28-29
Louvre, Paris 20-21
Mary Evans Picture Library, London 11, 17, 22-23, 24-25
Musée des Antquités Nationale, St Germain-en-Laye 22-23
Museo del Prado, Madrid 6
Museo Ostiense, Ostia 5, 22-23
National Library of Medicine, Bethesda, USA 30-31, 61
New York Academy of Medicine 28-29, 30-31, 34-35, 61
Nobel Foundation 5, 34-35, 36, 54-59, 61
Peabody Museum, Harvard University, Cambridge, USA 20-21
Peter Newark's Pictures 30-31
Playne Photographic 5, 10, 11, 12, 14, 15, 16, 18, 20-21, 22-23,
    24-25, 26-27, 28-29, 30-31, 32-33, 34-35, 36, 60, end papers
The Royal College of Physicians, London 28-29
The Royal College of Surgeons, London 30-31
The Science Photo Library, London 5, 30-31, 36
Semmelweiss Museum of Medical History, Budapest 30-31
Solo Syndication 36
The Stock Market, London 3, 5, 9, 34-35, 36, 53
The Wellcome Trust, London 5, 10, 11, 13, 16, 20-21, 22-23,
    24-25, 26-27, 28-29, 30-31, 32-33, 34-35, 36, 60
The Windsor Castle Royal Library, Great Britain 5, 26-27
World Health Organisation, Geneva 20-21
World Wide Photos, New York 61

While every effort has been made to trace copyright holders and
seek permission to use illustrative material, the publishers wish
to apologise for any inadvertent errors or ommissions and would
be glad to rectify these in future editions.

## 6
**Introduction**
By Professor Roy Porter
MA, PhD (cantab), FBA,
Hon.FRCP
Professor of the Social
History of Medicine
The Wellcome Institute
for the History of
Medicine

## 10
**Disease** and pestilence

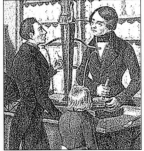

## 14
**Pharmacy** an ancient art

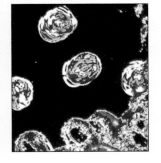

## 16
**Alternative** and
complementary medicine

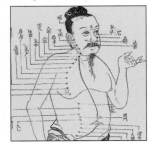

## 19
**How to use this book**
Explanation on how the
Timechart, and other
pages, work – to help
readers make the best
use of the book

## 20
**Timechart**
Prehistory to 0

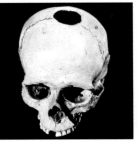

## 22
**Timechart**
0 to 1245 AD

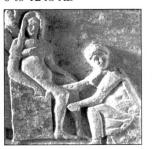

## 24
**Timechart**
1245 to 1470 AD

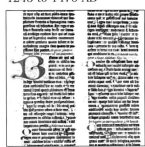

## 26
**Timechart**
1470 to 1580 AD

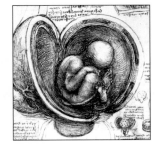

## 28
**Timechart**
1580 to 1690 AD

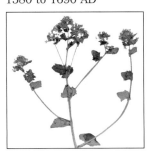

## 30
**Timechart**
1690 to 1780 AD

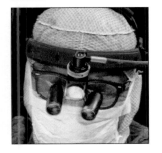

## 32
**Timechart**
1780 to 1855 AD

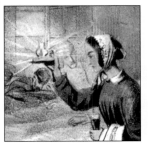

## 34
**Timechart**
1855 to 1955 AD

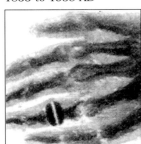

## 36
**Timechart**
1955 to 2000 AD

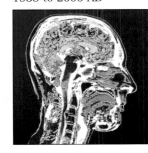

## 37
**Fact finder**
An index-style summary
of the information on the
Timechart to help locate
dates, people, nations
and events

## 53
**The future** What lies
ahead?

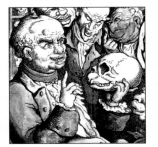

## 54
**Nobel prize winners**
in medicine, physics
and chemistry

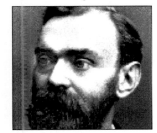

## 60
**Women** - their role as
doctors and the struggles
involved as they fought
their way to join the
medical profession

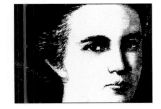

## 62
**Countries** a brief resumé
of events in medical
history as they occurred
in particular nations

## 68
**Bibliography** and further
reading: includes
Internet information, as
well as a variety of books
and works on many
aspects of medicine

## 72
**Museums** and
institutions: places to
discover more about the
history of medicine – a
selection from various
countries

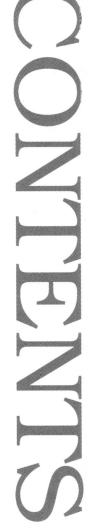

CONTENTS

# INTRODUCTION

by Roy Porter
Professor of
the Social History
of Medicine at the
The Wellcome Institute
for the History of
Medicine

Standing back and surveying the development of mankind on Earth, it could be said that virtually nothing has affected human history so much as disease. We have evolved in intimate connection with all manner of microscopic pathogens that have proved severe health risks. Above all, civilisation has had its disadvantages for human health, bringing with it a multitude of new diseases, associated with settlement, agriculture and animal husbandry.

Many of the worst diseases have arisen from proximity with animals. Cattle provided the pathogen pool with tuberculosis and viral poxes like smallpox. Pigs and ducks gave humans their influenzas, while horses brought rhinoviruses and hence the common cold. Measles - still killing a million children a year - is the result of canine distemper jumping between dogs or cattle and humans. Moreover, cats, dogs, ducks, hens, mice, rats and reptiles carry bacteria like *Salmonella*, leading to fatal human infections such as hepatitis, whooping cough and diphtheria. Current fears over the relationship between bovine spongiform encephalopathy (BSE), and the human Creuzfeld-Jacob Disease (CJD) remind us how vulnerable mankind has always been to infections transferred from animals.

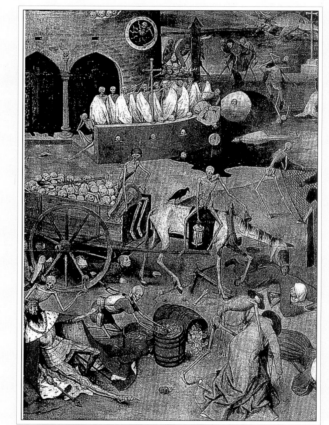

The city, hub of civilisation, has become the nucleus of disease. The towns of Renaissance Europe were riddled with typhus, typhoid and plague. The industrial cities of the nineteenth century harboured tuberculosis, the 'white plague'. Whilst mankind was at the the hunter-gatherer stage, disease was insignificant. With the coming of civilisation, cities and the world population explosion which has occurred over the last ten thousand years, epidemics and pandemics have come to play a major part on the stage of world history.

Many of the turning-points in human affairs can be put down less to the best-laid plans of men than to misadventures with micro-organisms. For example, the collapse of the feudal system in the Middle Ages was in large measure the result of the devastating invasion of Europe by bubonic plague. In the 1340s the Black Death killed up to one third of Europe's entire population, a calamity on a scale unimaginable nowadays except in the context of nuclear war.

Or take the conquest of the New World by the Old, initiated by Columbus's voyage across the Atlantic in search of the 'Indies' in 1492. The victory was due to less to the guns or guile of the *Conquistadores* that to the fact that the Spanish invaders were carrying with them the pathogens of disease to which *they* had some acquired immunity but to which New World natives had none at all. It is believed that by 1600 up to ninety per cent of the American indians had died in successive disease onslaughts, and the fabric of native life fell to pieces. It was thus disease rather than military might which vanquished the New World. Ironically, Columbus's men may have brought back with them one New World disease – that is, syphilis – which was to prove the scourge of Europe, colouring the gloomy religious and artistic culture of the time.

Disease, in other words, has played a major part in human history, albeit one which most historians have generally ignored or down-played. Humans have, of course, attempted to fight back – to prevent and, above all, to master disease through a variety of means including religion and magic, but above all, medicine. Healing has been practised throughout recorded time. There is archeological evidence, from as far afield as France, South America and the Pacific, that as early as 3000 BC trephining or trepanning was being performed, cutting a small hole in the skull with a flint, presumably to allow the escape of evil spirits. Our first written records of medicine as an art and practice come from Mesopotamia and Egypt. Medicine as a rational science developed in that 'Greek miracle' erupting around the Eastern Mediterranean from around 500 BC. Hippocrates, the so-called 'father of medicine', was an older contemporary of Plato.

What this time-chart presentation, juxtaposing the history of disease and the development of medicine, makes so clear is that the battle was for long wholly

procedures, like bloodletting, were almost certainly positively harmful. It is often said, not entirely facetiously, that it wasn't until after 1900 that a visit to the doctor was likely to leave you in a better state of health. In surgery, for example, it was only in the nineteenth century that it became possible to perform any ambitious surgical interventions, for example opening up

*Disease, in other words, has played a major part in human history, albeit one which most historians have generally ignored or down-played.*

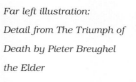

*Far left illustration: Detail from The Triumph of Death by Pieter Breughel the Elder*

*Left illustration: Operating theatre at Jefferson Medical College, Philadelphia. Watched by students at the University of Pennsylvania, D. Hayes Agnew and his theatre staff perform an operation in about 1870*

unequal. Disease was rampant and medicine, however worthy, was for thousands of years a weak reed, ineffectual in saving the lives of those afflicted or at getting to grips with the real understanding of disease and its causes.

For most of the history of mankind, the story of medicine has been, at best, one of very slow and partial improvements in the understanding of the cause and cure of disorders. The workings of the human body in sickness and in health began to make considerable strides from the Renaissance onwards with the rise of anatomy, physiology and pathology, but, in the short term, those advances did little to restore the health of the sick. Only recently have scientists and doctors developed the skills, tools, techniques and drugs which reliably save lives. Certain traditional medical

the stomach or the chest. Until then, even attempts to set compound fractures often proved fatal, since lethal infections would set in. Only in the twentieth century have we acquired drugs which are truly effective in fighting disease - the sulpha drugs pioneered in the 1930s and the antibiotics which came in during the Second World War. This time-chart history shows very clearly how unequal the warfare between microbes and man has been through most of history.

The other thing visible at a glance by this time-chart presentation is the great complexity of medicine. There are some human human endeavours – mathematics, for example, or perhaps theoretical physics – in which progress occurs as a result of the brilliant intuitions or experiments of a tiny elite of geniuses, working largely in their heads. Medicine, however, is

*What this time-chart presentation, juxtaposing the history of disease and the development of medicine, makes so clear is that the battle was for long wholly unequal.*

*Within medicine, as the charts indicate, one development triggers another in a kind of (generally unplanned) chain-reaction.*

not like that at all. Medicine requires the confluence and cooperation of all manner of different activities, occupations and crafts, and the alliance of theoretical knowledge with practical skill.

The improvements in medicine in the Victorian era, for instance, depended upon the concatenation of multiple developments occurring on a broad front. Hospitals had to emerge as locations where, at one and the same time, sufferers were treated, students were taught their trade, and the serried ranks of the

trial towns. And, not least, the state had increasingly to intervene to regulate and promote health and fund the treatment of the sick. All these diverse factors had to be present for medical progress to occur.

Within medicine, as the charts indicate, one development triggers another in a kind of (generally unplanned) chain-reaction. Take surgery. Before the nineteenth century, the 'cutter's art' was stymied by two key obstacles: pain and infection. Luckily, around 1800, the chemist Humphry Davy, pioneer-

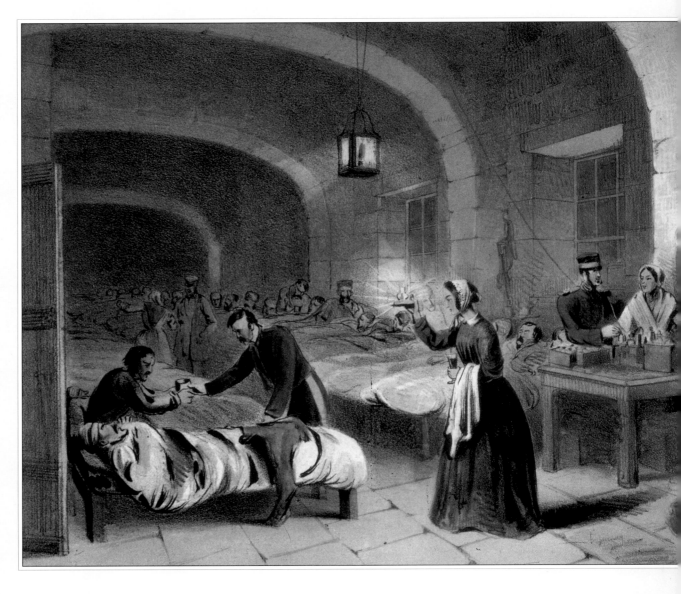

*Florence Nightingale on her rounds at the field hospital in Scutari. She reduced the Crimean War hospital death rate from 42% to 2%*

*The other thing visible at a glance by this time-chart presentation is the great complexity of medicine.*

sick could stimulate systematic study of disease itself (in the last resort, through the conduct of post mortems in the morgue). Universities had to be reformed, so as to become powerhouses of new basic sciences – biology, chemistry, microscopy, and housing the specialised laboratories which stimulated so many discoveries. The medical professional had to be reformed, ensuring high-quality training and the elimination of quackery. Nursing had to be professionalised. A new type of public health had to be created to control the 'filth diseases' rampant in indus-

ing the science of gas chemistry, experimented with nitrous oxide (laughing gas) and discovered its anaesthetising properties. During the next generation, that gas, along with ether and chloroform, began to be tried out in America. Ether was used surgically in Paris and in London in December 1846 – the Scots-born Robert Liston amputated a diseased thigh from a patient under ether, pronouncing 'This Yankee dodge, gentlemen, beats mesmerism hollow'; – 'Hail Happy Hour! We Have Conquered Pain!' sang the newspaper headlines. And then the key event came on 7 April 1853: Queen Victoria took chloroform for the birth of Prince Leopold. 'The effect was soothing, quieting and delightful beyond measure,' Her Majesty recorded in her journal.

Meanwhile, microscopists were establishing how inflammation, infection and putrefaction were related to the micro-organisms revealed squirming under their lenses. This gave surgeons a clue as to why so many of their patients died of post-operative sepsis. Effective antiseptic techniques were then pioneered

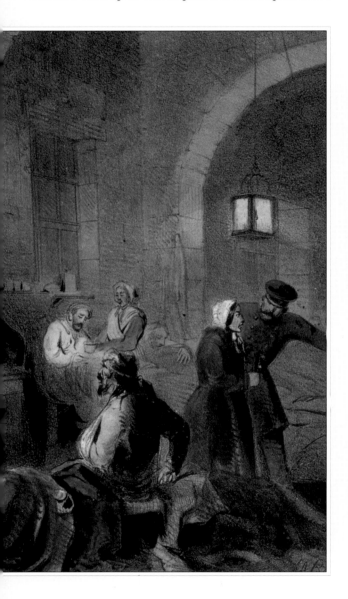

in the 1860s in Glasgow by Joseph Lister. Thereafter it became possible to open up the human body, not just *painlessly* but *safely*. The door had been opened to modern surgery.

It can thus be seen that medicine is an infinitely complex jigsaw-puzzle in which everything is interlocking. And, historically, the links between events have often been complicated, oblique and totally unpredictable. The value of the time-charts presentation is that such connections are made visible at a glance.

The flow of time is also made clear: the great stream of biological evolution itself, lethal pandemics, large-scale social change, and the parts played by individual pioneers, from Hippocrates, through Vesalius, up to Pasteur and the doctors and scientists alive today.

The history of medicine is a heroic story, in so far as it has been a gallant fight against Death. But it has been a far from complete triumph, For millennia, disease humbled the powers of the doctors, and it would be foolishly short-sighted of us nowadays - however tremendous the achievements of recent medical science – to this that this situation has irrevocably

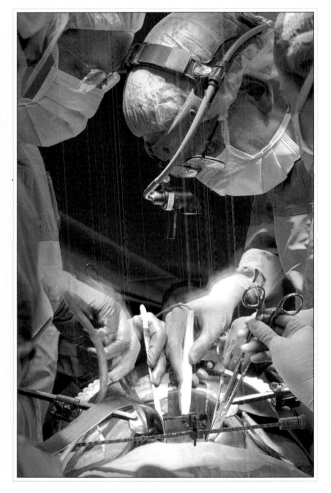

changed. Evolutionary theory teaches us the law of the survival of the fittest. Bacteria and viruses have always shown themselves to be survivors. The sage of medicine is an ongoing struggle.

**Roy S Porter**
MA, PhD (cantab), FBA, Hon.FRCP
Professor of the Social History of Medicine
The Wellcome Institute for the History of Medicine
London July 1999

*The value of the time-charts presentation is that such connections are made visible at a glance. The flow of time is also made clear: the great stream of biological evolution itself, lethal pandemics, large-scale social change, and the parts played by individual pioneers, from Hippocrates, through Vesalius, up to Pasteur and the doctors and scientists alive today*

*Modern surgery encompasses the learning of centuries and has made astounding progress in recent years – but disease is still ever-prevalent.*

# DISEASE

**AND PESTILENCE**

W e cannot be sure exactly which diseases ravaged early prehistoric man but once the written recording of events began, those diseases which killed large numbers of the population have been noted appropriately.

The patterns have changed – with each age and community subject to the weaknesses of its own social structure, hygiene, and areas of ignorance. But prevention or cure has not necessarily advanced hand in hand with greater knowledge. And even as treatment has improved and certain diseases checked to some degree, so new ones seem to emerge to confound the scientists.

The number of diseases that have swept through communities during the history of mankind is vast. Within the confines of this short account, there is only space to look briefly at a few. However, the Bibliography refers to several books that can provide much more information for those who wish to know more.

## Leprosy

The leprosy bacillus was not discovered until 1873, but had been busy causing disease and great fear of infection throughout man's history. In 600 BC leprosy was recorded in India. Biblical leprosy is a form of 'uncleanness' and in all probability has no connection with the disease of that name. Another translation error resulted in the further complication of *elephantiasis graecorum* (leprory) becoming known as *lepra arabum*. The arabs themselves recognised that elephantaisis was a different disease.

There are some who believe that leprosy was brought back from the East by the Crusaders to Europe but, whatever lay behind its appearance, leprosy was prevalent throughout the Middle Ages. By that time the clergy were seen as the means of salvation and healing.

However, sufferers were still isolated from the rest of the community, and often banned from towns altogether. From about the year 1000 lepers were excluded from normal society. Even in recent times the victims have been cut off from normal life. For example, Spinalonga, an island close to Crete, housed Greek lepers as recently as 1957.

For various reasons, leprosy declined in the later Middle Ages. Much later on, Armaeur Hansen studied the disease in Bergen Norway and he succeeded in isolating the leprosy bacteria in 1873. The first International Conference on the subject was held in Berlin in 1893 and in 1921 the British established ninety-four leprosy asylums in India.

Nowadays leprosy can be treated with chemotherapy. It no longer carries its certain threat of disfigurement and slow painful death.

*Right:*
*Initially, the concept of an injection derived from cowpox created some fear and ridicule – as this contemporary cartoon shows*

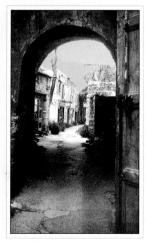

*Spinalonga, the leper island near Crete*

## Smallpox

It is possible that smallpox was rampant in 10,000 BC and it seemsto have occurred in Ancient Egypt. The mummy of Pharoah Rameses V (which dates back to 1160 BC) shows typical pockmarks.

In the tenth century Persian physician, Rhazes, described the disease, distinguishing it from measles.

There was a veritable plague of smallpox which devastated Europe in 1693 to 1694 when England's young Queen Mary 11 died as one of its victims. There were outbreaks in New England too and smallpox decimated the North American Indian tribes.

The Chinese inoculated against smallpox, placing pus from a mild case into a scratch on a healthy person. The Turks used a similar technique which was noted by Lady Mary Wortley Montagu (wife to the British Ambassador in Turkey in the early eighteenth century). She brought the notion back with her to Britain where its value was recognised and inoculation instigated – though at some risk to the first 'guinea pigs' as the live virus, albeit selected from mild cases, could occasionally turn out to be a virulent strain.

Later this procedure was made safer by Edward Jenner in 1798 when he discovered that milkmaids who

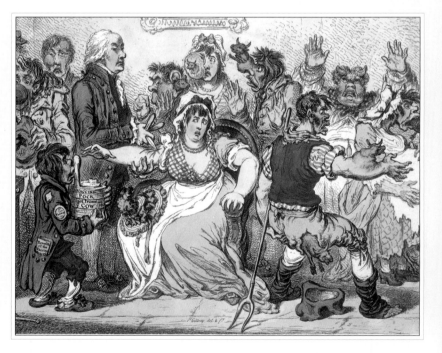

had contracted cowpox developed resistance to smallpox. He used cowpox in his new-fangled 'vaccinations' which soon became very popular and considerably reduced the presence of smallpox in Britain.

In 1967 smallpox was still a major threat but as vaccinations spread all around the world its impact grew less and less until in 1980 the World Health Organisation was able to announce that it had been completely eradicated.

## Plague

Rat-borne plague is first thought to have emerged from the Himalayan borderlands between India and China. Pestilence struck the Roman Empire between AD 165 and 180 and may have been a mix of several diseases the soldiers carried back with them from Mesopotamia but some sources claim it was predominantly smallpox. Then there was a second wave of pestilence, along with measles, in 251-266. At its height this outbreak is believed to have killed 5,000 people a day in Rome.

The Plague of Justinian struck in 542 and the appearance of large buboes as swollen lymph nodes were clearly recorded. These can be egg-sized but may have swollen to the size of a apple. At any rate, Procopius reported that plague killed 10,000 people a day in Constantinople.

There were several plague outbreaks in Britain – one of which was clearly described by the Venerable Bede in 664.

Bubonic plague spread right across the world in the Middle Ages, carried, in the first instance, by fleas on the black rats that infested ships. Plague can be spread from person to person (by the bacteria in the coughs and sneezes of its human victims) when it reaches the lungs and causes

pneumonic plague. It may have been called the Black Death because of its symptoms: dark swollen lymph glands or simply because black is associated with horror. Bubonic plague raged between 1347 and 1351 killing some 75 million people – between 25 and 50 per cent of the population in afflicted areas of Europe and the Middle East.

Quarantine was introduced by the Venetians at Ragusa in 1377. In some ports ships had to wait forty

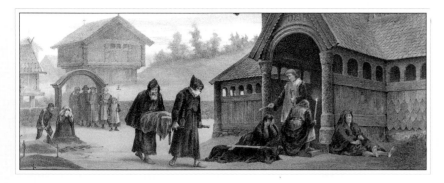

days (*quaranta* being Italian for forty) before disembarkation was allowed.

During the fifteenth, sixteenth and seventeenth centuries, plague recurred throughout Europe. It was endemic in England following the Black Death but the first cases of the Great Plague appeared in London in 1664; it reached its peak in 1665 and killed a huge proportion of London's population (about 15 per cent – some 80,000 people). At risk of spreading the disease, many fled the city. The dead were collected daily and taken away in handcarts to mass graves dug outside the city walls.

The disease spread widely over the country but then its virulence seemed suddenly to subside. The Great Fire of London is often attributed with having killed the bacteria but in fact it appears that it had 'run its course' in other parts of the country as well – and its impact lessened in mainland Europe too.

By the 1790s the Chinese were commenting on the association of the appearance of numbers of dying rats with the disease. None the less, the ebb and flow of plague remains a mystery and may be associated with changing trade routes and density of rat populations. Several twentieth-century outbreaks indicate that plague is still perhaps only 'waiting in the wings'!

### Cholera

At one time cholera was confined to the East and still recurs annually as an epidemic in India. It was studied by Jacobus Bontius from Holland in the Dutch East Indies in 1627 who described it accurately in 1642.

It spread from India to China where an outbreak in 1669 lead to its fully-fledged introduction into the Western World. There it flourished in towns and cities for the next two centuries or so, the ideal conditions for its spread to be found in these industrialised areas with crowded housing and poor sanitation. In 1831-2 cholera killed 5,000 in London and many thousands worldwide. Then another 50,000 succumbed in 1849-50. It was prevalent in the USA by 1836-1838 and during the American Ciivil War some 50,000 died.

Queen Victoria's physician, John Snow, noted during an outbreak in

Soho in 1854 that cases centred around the Broad Street water pump. Local brewery workers who rarely drank water or those drawing water from a different pump did not appear to catch cholera. By simply organis-

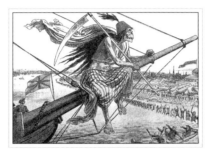

ing the removal of the Broad Street pump handle, Snow stopped the outbreak; there were no more new cases. Snow had proved that the disease spread through contaminated drinking water.

Nowadays it is largely kept at bay because of good standards of sanitation and water purification but cholera still occurs regularly in the Far East and where primitive living conditions prevail.

### Typhoid

Typhoid symptoms are varied and not necessarily specific to typhoid alone so it is difficult to ascertain its history precisely. Although a member of the salmonella family, typhoid is purely a human disease and is generally transmitted via polluted water and poor sanitation.

In the eighteenth century there was a general belief that many diseases, including typhoid, were spread through filth and foul air. William Budd argued in 1839 that although typhoid was certainly due to insanitary conditions it was not just 'in the air' but a contagious infection carried from one person to another. When in 1847 he investigated one outbreak amongst students who had used a common well his theories were further substantiated.

Budd also distinguished typhoid from typhus which is spread by human lice.

In 1901 Robert Koch discovered that typhoid could be transmitted by seemingly healthy carriers. One such was 'Typhoid Mary' an American–

Irish cook in Long Island who was actually kept in jail for three years to prevent her coming into contact with the general public. She is known to have caused at least forty-seven cases of typhoid and three deaths.

Vaccinations were used during the First World War and prevented the troops from being ravaged by the disease, despite their dreadful living conditions. Now antibiotics and greatly improved hygiene mean that typhoid has virtually disappeared from developed countries but there still remain some 15 million cases of typhoid and a million deaths a year.

In the USA in 1900 there was annual death rate of 30 per 100,000 population. In 1960 the total number of deaths was only twenty-one.

### Tuberculosis

Prior to pasteurisation, TB was sometimes transmitted to humans from cows through contaminated milk but the bacilli are more generally passed from human to human by being carried in airborne droplets.

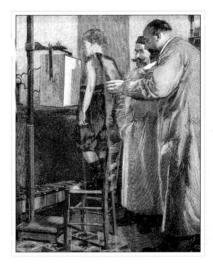

Historically, a form of tuberculosis has been described under the term 'scrofula' which denoted a number of diseases that caused swollen glands. This was 'The King's Evil' since it was believed that a royal touch could cure the disease.

During the nineteenth century reports suggest that a vast proportion of the British population suffered from the disease including a good number of children but few died from a bovine infection. It was the pulmonary TB – rife in the eighteenth and nineteenth centuries and then called 'consumption' – that was lethal. The mortality rates were very high and it was the leading cause of death in European and American cities in the nineteenth century.

Bacteriologist Robert Koch identified the bacillus in the 1880s but it was not until the 1920s that the BCG vaccine began to be used widely.

Vaccination (although often controversial) and understanding of

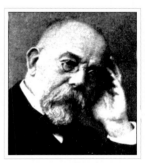

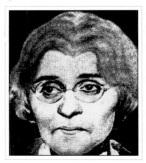

hygiene have reduced the impact of the disease in the developed world but it still appears hand in hand with poverty and in races or territories where there has been no previous exposure. Because of their diminished immunity, AIDS victims are highly susceptible to the bacillus.

## Syphilis

Syphilis or the 'Pox' is one of several venereal diseases and it is sometimes difficult to ascertain which particular disease is being referred to in the earliest historical records.

It was certainly present in a mild form in Europe before 1492 but seems to have suddenly become deadly after Christopher Columbus's discovery of the Americas. It may be that an American strain returned with his crew or crossed with the European form, although this theory is now disputed. Perhaps the disease mutated in some way. Whatever the cause, a virulent outbreak spread across the face of Europe in 1493-94 and was a veritable plague until about 1530 – and it has recurred ever since.

*Once Columbus had landed in America the route was opened up for the exchange of diseases. Populations not previously exposed to a disease were particularly susceptible and, as the Spaniards arrived, so measles stuck in places like Brazil and Mexico*

breaks that have become world-wide pandemics and exacted a heavy death toll. Hippocrates described an epidemic in the 5th century BC that may have been influenza. There was certainly one clearly described in 1610.

Russian flu in 1781-2 swept over Europe from the east and again in 1889 – when it reached all the populated continents and killed about 250,000 in Europe.

Generally sweeping universally, influenza was so-named because eighteenth-century Italian physicians believed its spread was *influenced* by the stars.

In 1918 almost the entire northern hemisphere was blanketed by the disease in a single month; it became one of the most severe killer diseases in history. Latest examinations of the records estimate that some 30 million may have died in a matter of a few months, with some fifty times that figure being taken ill. 548,000 died in the USA and perhaps as many as 20 million in India in this most catastrophic of outbreaks. The death toll in one year was higher than that of the entire First World War.

known to decimate races, adults and children alike, in places such as Mexico, the Fiji islands and Alaska where previously unexposed and therefore vulnerable victims have succumbed in great numbers.

Its recorded history does not begin until the 10th century when the Muslim physician Rhazes described it and then a century later, Avicenna, a Persian scientist, postulated that the rash was due to residual menstrual blood from the mother.

By the sixteenth and seventeenth centuries, physicians were better equipped to distinguish between measles and scarlet fever. Earlier confusion had occurred because there was a less 'clinical' approach and physicians tended to analyse the types of people susceptible to particular diseases rather than concentrating on the close inspection of specific symptoms and signs.

It was not until the nineteenth century that outbreaks in colonies and settlements created a catastrophic death toll. The deaths were in part due to the disease and its complications but also to exhaustion and starvation because when whole communities were taken ill *en masse*, there was no-one to care for the young, sick or elderly.

During a severe outbreak in the Faeroes in 1846 when 6,100 of the population of 7,864 contracted measles, Peter Ludwig Panum of Denmark conducted a thorough research into the pattern of the disease. This proved that once the distinctive measles rash appeared, the contagious 'flu-like' stage had already been passed and so quarantine was ineffective

Ever a disease of war, spread by the mobilisation of soldiers and the close confines of military camps, from the American Civil War to World War One, it became clear to the various military medical authorities, that the best protection was still exposure in childhood until such time as vaccines became available. A vaccine created from modified live measles virus has been in use widely since the 1960s and considerably lessened the impact of measles, and its side effects as a disease of childhood.

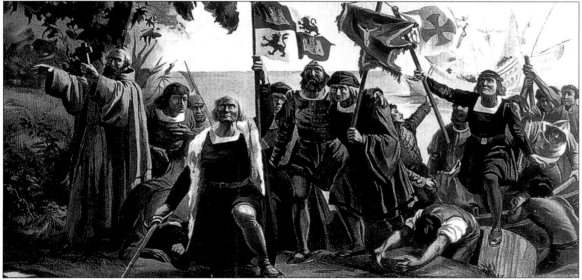

It was treated variously with substances such as mercury and guaiacum (from a Columbian timber) – and generally regarded as a symbol of immorality and vice by the end of the eighteenth century.

The use of penicillin and antibiotics mean that although the disease is still omnipresent, deaths from syphilis have greatly diminished since the 1940s.

## Influenza

Spread by a virus, influenza is highly contagious but is often only of brief duration and – unless respiratory complications set in – is rarely fatal. Particularly susceptible are the very young and the old who are most likely to develop associated bronchitis or pneumonia but there have been out-

*Right:*
*Mosquito: it is the female whose bite carries the malaria micro-organism*

In the 1930s new electron microscopes enabled scientists to photograph and better distinguish the various strains of the virus and at last vaccines were able to be developed. There was an epidemic of Asian influenza in 1957 which began in China and then circled the globe, becoming more virulent as it did so, with respiratory complications increasing by the time it reached America. However, the prompt and widespread use of the specific flu vaccine ahead of the arrival of the disease reduced its severity and lessened mortality rates in the States.

## Measles

Measles is primarily a childhood disease but it does not entirely belong to the nursery, of course, and has been

## Malaria

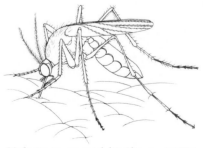

Malaria is caused by the parasitic protozoa, *Plasmodium*, which is carried by the females of certain mosquito species and injected into humans

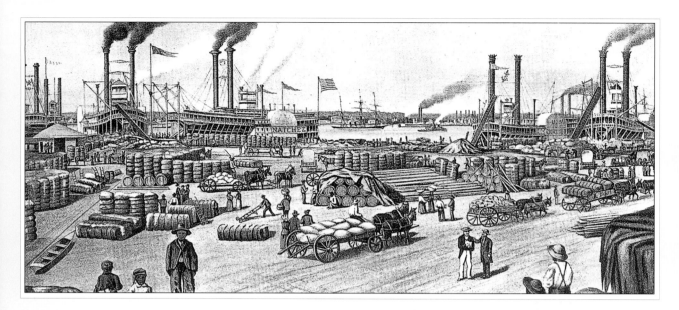

*Outbreaks of yellow fever repeatedly spread from tropical regions through ports such as New Orleans (here shown as it was in 1884)*

when bitten by these insects. It is still rife in tropical Africa, Asia and Central and South America.

Malaria leaves no marks on bones so it is hard to trace its history in ancient times. We do know that it has been ubiquitous in warm climates for centuries and in 2700 BC a medical book *Nei Ching* described the swollen spleen and cycle of fever that would seem to be typical of malaria. In 1600 BC Sumerian and Vedic writing show malaria was prevalent then.

Several times malaria battered the defences of the Roman Empire more powerfully than any military force had done.

There were severe outbreaks in Columbia in 1493. In 1630 the Countess of Chinchón was treated with an infusion from the bark of a Peruvian tree now named after her and its active ingredient, quinine, has since been used universally for treating cases of malaria.

Although long associated with marshy areas and with several nineteenth-century investigators linking it to parasites, malaria's association with the mosquito was not properly understood until the beginning of the twentieth century.

In the twentieth century, with its increasing scientific 'manipulation' of the natural world, it had been believed that the draining of marshy areas and the use of DDT on stagnant water would eradicate most of the malaria-carrying mosquitoes and therefore the disease itself but the subsequent withdrawal of DDT and the development of resistant species has meant that malaria is still very much in evidence.

## Yellow fever

In the jungle areas of Africa and America, this was long regarded as a non-lethal disease of childhood – as indeed it was until the arrival of non-immune Europeans into these parts of the world. The slave trade in turn introduced Yellow Fever to new areas

and unprotected victims. Carried by mosquitoes through a chain of insect-monkey-insect or insect-man-insect, the disease is caused by a flavivirus and attacks the liver, causing severe yellow jaundice – hence the name Yellow Fever

After its first appearance in Barbados in 1647 it spread through American ports and into some European ports, including Lisbon, Barcelona and Swansea. Its impact in the Caribbean area was fearsome. In 1655, of 1,500 French soldiers in St Lucia, only eighty-nine survived. In time ships had to fly the warning Yellow Jack flag if stricken and in the 1850s there were several severe outbreaks in New Orleans.

As was the case with a number of diseases then, many physicians believed that Yellow Fever was an illness that arose from the fetid air in streets where dead animals lay rotting and human waste accumulated to create horrid vapours.

Eventually (following Ronald Ross's researches in malaria) in 1899 Walter Reed, an American physician, suggested that Yellow Fever was also carried by mosquitoes. Carlos Finlay, a physician in Cuba, had proposed a similar notion in the 1880s but he transferred mosquitoes fed on yellow fever patients to uninfected volunteers after only three to five days – t oo short a time for the virus to have fully developed in the carrier so had been unable to prove his theories.

In due course, volunteer soldiers were split into two groups. One set was exposed to the soiled bedding and clothing of yellow fever victims; the second set to mosquitoes known to have already bitten yellow fever patients. Only those unfortunates in the second group contracted the disease so the mosquito agency was established. The Reed Commission also established that yellow fever was caused by a virus.

In Havana and the Panama Canal area, William Crawford Gorgas spearheaded the control of mosqui-

toes through swamp drainage, oiling of the breeding sites, and using insecticides and screening sick rooms. By the 1930s a vaccine had been created. Yellow Fever slithered back to the confines of the jungle but is not entirely defeated. It still flares up now and then in tropical cities.

## AIDS

AIDS is caused by the HIV virus. It is unaffected by antibiotics and is as yet incurable. Aids does not kill directly but prevents the body's defence systems from killing other bacteria and viruses – so victims are unable to defend themselves against subsequent diseases.

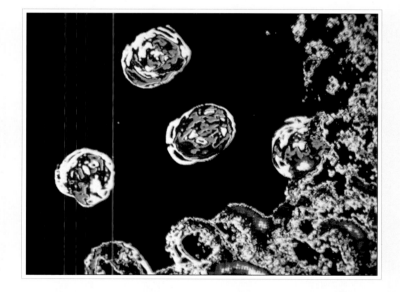

*AIDS virus*

It emerged in Central Africa as new highways opened up routes into the rain forests, linking hitherto isolated areas with the rest of the world. Soon Aids spread to Western Europe and America where it was first recognised in Los Angeles and New York in 1981. The World Health Organisation estimates that 5 to 10 million people are infected with the HIV virus and that it is rapidly increasing its spread all over the world.

# PHARMACY

**AN
ANCIENT
ART**

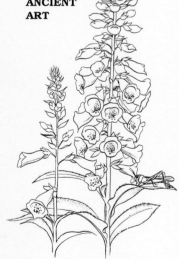

Digitalis, from foxgloves, had long
been used as a secret ingredient
of herbal cures. In 1785 William
Withering made public its use for
treating dropsy. It is still used
today for heart conditions

Right:
The Apothecary's Shop by Pietro
Longhi. As well as dispensing
drugs, apothecaries sometimes
acted as dentists

**P**harmacy is the science of preparing and using drugs. From time immemorial the skills of pharmacy have involved the cultivation of plants that have continually been used as a major source of drugs. Minerals and animal products have also been implemented – and, more recently, the list has included synthesised chemical compounds.

This is an ancient art, practised in one form or another since primitive man first extracted juice from plants to help healing or to soothe wounds. There are many references in the Bible to ointments and medications. Moreover, many of the products used at the time of the Ancient Greeks, and some from as long ago as Ancient Egypt (like the castor oil plant) still prove to have useful properties today.

However, many very strange concoctions were also employed by the Ancients and included such exotic ingredients as crocodile droppings, lapis lazuli, opium, hemlock potions, pounded pine, prunes, wine dregs, lizard dung, sulphur, cow and goat milk, honey and wax, lion fat, castor, human and dog excrement, cattle urine and poppy seeds in beer.

## Physician and apothecary

The role of the pharmacist was at one time undertaken by the healers themselves, who prepared their own medications but in due course the areas of responsibility became separate. Even the physician-priests of Egypt were divided into two types: there were those who tended the sick and those who remained in the temples to prepare remedies for the patients. Egyptian prescriptions were made up in proportion to fractions based on the eye of Horus. The Hearst Papyrus (c. 1550 BC) is inscribed with some 250 prescriptions.)

According to legend, Asclepius (who was the Greek god of healing) delegated the duty of compounding his remedies to his daughter, Hygieia, the goddess of health – who thence became his apothecary.

The Arabian influence in Europe during the eighth century AD further separated the role of pharmacist and physician. Then, during the Middle Ages in Europe, there was a distinct separation between the roles of the physician and apothecary. The physician prescribed whilst the apothecary supplied and dispensed medicines. The physician dealt with the patient.

## Herbals

In the first century AD the first Western herbal was written by a Greek army surgeon, Dioscorides, and was a materia medica.

The Chinese have a long record of using drugs, with books on roots and herbs appearing as early as the third millennium BC when the legendary Shen Nong listed some 365 drugs, and medicinal herbs.

Juliana Anicia, daughter of a Roman emperor, put together one of the earliest herbals before AD 512 while John Gerard compiled much herbal lore into his Herball, published in 1597 – with a new improved edition in 1653.

Nicholas Culpeper published his famous Herbal in 1653 and it has remained in print ever since.

The World Health Organisation of the United Nations began publishing the Pharmacopoeia Internationalis in the early 1950s.

## Growing knowledge

Arab medical practitioners had accumulated an enormous store of infor-

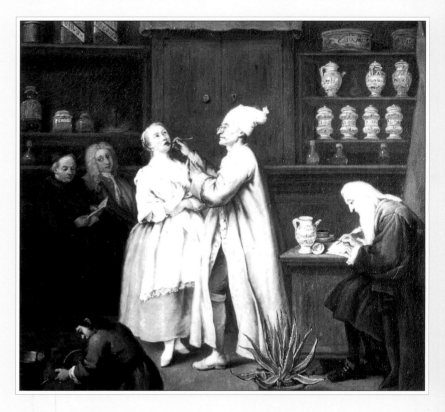

mation about herbs and medicines. Rhazes (864 - 925), the Persian physician and medical author, introduced many new herbs to the Western world. Later, the Normans established 'spicers' into the households of places that they conquered, including Great Britain. The spicer's role was to add the right spices to improve or disguise the dubious flavour of the preserved winter meat. In time, the role of these spicers evolved into that of the herbalist and apothecary.

Medieval monks grew herb gardens in order to have the vital ingredients at hand to prepare their cures. Apothecaries also became skilled specialists.

## The role of women

In feudal times the lady of the manor was often deemed responsible for the health of the family and those who served them – and so accumulated knowledge that was passed on from mother to daughter: many effective herbal remedies were developed and dispensed by her ladyship to help the sick. She would grow the herbs in her garden and these included sage, mint hyssop, thyme, parsley, marjoram and bay.

There were many wise old women, midwives, and faith healers – who all prescribed herbs. Much of this knowledge was passed on orally except among the more educated wise women, the nuns and lay sisters, who kept records of their herbal cures.

Sadly, during the Middle Ages and right up until the eighteenth century, there was a great fear of black magic and witchcraft and some of the wise women, despite the fact that their knowledge and cures were helping their neighbours, were regarded with suspicion: the better their remedies the more likely these were to be seen as spells so the unfortunate women were sometimes regarded as evil and persecuted.

## Vipers and toads

There was a great trade in vipers in the Middle Ages as their blood, once dried, was the major ingredient of theriac, an important drug used from the eleventh to the seventeenth century. It was supposed to cure all manner of things, including syphilis and plague. (Today Russell's viper venom is used to help haemophiliac blood to clot.)

Other popular drugs included unicorn horn (which was taken from narwhal whale tusks) and toad stones. These were supposedly extracted from a toad's head!

## A changing world

The discoveries of the Americas and wider exploration of the world in general, and its resources, led in turn to the discovery of new plants and fresh sources of herbs and drugs. However it seems that these new exciting possibilities were not tapped as fully as they might have been and, although some plant substances were imported, many potentially useful drugs were not introduced into Europe from the New World.

Meanwhile, a law enacted by the city council of Bruges in 1683 forbade physicians to prepare medications for their patients. This was now stipulated to be the prerogative of the pharmacist only.

In America, Benjamin Franklin, founder and first president of the Pennsylvania Hospital appointed an apothecary to the hospital and this underlined the two separate 'entities' of physician and pharmacist.

## Chemistry

Whilst the natural world provided sufficient ingredients for the herbalist in the Middle Ages, as more towns sprang up and spread, meadows and forest vanished and it became necessary to produce more drugs for an increasing urban population from diminishing resources.

Apothecaries' shops were established, each covering its own district, to supply local needs. Plants were bought in from the countryside and foreign ingredients and medicines imported from further afield.

Meanwhile, the work and study of alchemists (whose aim was to turn base substances into gold) contributed much to the knowledge of the time. In practical terms, they perfected the techniques of distillation and the isolation of acids, alcohol and metals and, in their approaches to research, exposed new concepts in chemistry, opening up routes of knowledge that would eventually lead to biochemistry and chemotherapy.

As understanding of chemistry grew and the constituent elements of the plants used was better understood, so pharmacy took on a more scientific role. Chemical compounds and formulae were appreciated and implemented.

## Theophrastus Philippus Aureolus Parcelsus

Paracelsus (1493-1541) was a physician from Switzerland whose theories encouraged the search for the active constituents of medicinal plants and promoted chemical remedies and the more specific application of appropriate drugs. He also investigated painkillers. Paracelsus helped to improve and reform pharmaceutical practice and increase understanding of chemistry. In due course, in Britain, pharmacists and druggists replaced the apothecary (who became a medical practitioner), drugs began to be manufactured and advertised and an ever-expanding new industry was launched – the first proprietary pharmaceutical products appearing in the 1890s.

## The Quack

Since people who are ill, incapacitated, or in pain are always eager to try a new remedy – and are generally willing to part with money in order to do so – throughout history there have always been those eager to exploit the susceptibilities of these unfortunates and their relatives. Sellers of medicines would appear at fairs and, especially in the United States, toured in covered wagons to proffer their wares. Fear of a dread disease encouraged the onlookers to buy drugs to cure syphilis, tuberculosis, infertility and the like.

Not all touring quacks were complete charlatans and the occasional one may have helped to improve the lives of his or her customers, if only by the placebo effect. Bottles of various tonics were offered and while some may indeed have been genuine herbal cures, most were of no real medicinal value. There was often a good deal of showmanship and trickery involved, with wildly exaggerated claims made for the products – many of which contained alcohol as a solvent and so certainly had an effect of some kind on the user!

New discoveries, such as electricity and radium, were supposedly incorporated into some of the nostrums or implements and the gullible were lured into parting with their cash for cures, means of rejuvenation, for aphrodisiacs, to grow more hair or to prevent its turning grey!

Licensing, legislation against unauthorised or unqualified practitioners, controls on unsubstantiated claims for products and the registration of new drugs and products has limited the impact of quackery today but there are still many cases of exploitation, in one form or another – and probably always will be!

## Education

Pharmacists had initially trained as apprentices, learning their skills from an expert, practising instructor over a long period of time 'on the job' – but the first college of pharmacy was founded in the United States in 1821. It is now known as the Philadelphia College of Pharmacy and Science.

Other institutes and colleges were established soon after in the United States, Great Britain, and continental Europe.

The Pharmaceutical Society of Great Britain was established in 1841 and the American Pharmaceutical Association was established in 1852.

The Fédération Internationale Pharmaceutique was founded in 1910 and is supported by over fifty national societies.

## The twentieth century

The discovery and use of new drug substances in the twentieth century has added to the responsibilities of the pharmacist in a fast-changing medical environment. The pharmacist continues, however, to fulfil the role accepted through the centuries – to meet the physician's requirements, to provide qualified advice and information; to formulate the correct medicines, store the necessary stocks and ingredients, and to provide correct dosages. It is also his or her responsibility to ensure the medicinal products used are of the best quality.

Pharmacists today have to prepare a wide range of tablets, capsules, syrups and solutions, as well as understanding an ever-expanding range of proprietary products. Their role is still to fulfil the prescriptions set out by doctors, physicians, dentists, and veterinarians but they may be a great source of advice and knowledge too.

Colleges of pharmacy now operate in most developed countries of the world, with full courses of instruction taking at least five years to complete and embracing many related sciences. Simultaneously, pharmacy laws have evolved to ensure safety is maintained and these include regulations for the practice of pharmacy, the sale of poisons, the dispensing of narcotics, and the labelling and sale of dangerous drugs.

All new products have to be screened and registered. Today the licensing systems for new medicinal products in Europe and North America demand extensive investigation, the testing of products in the laboratory and thorough clinical trials to establish their efficacy and safety.

## Herbs and cures used for centuries

Digitalis from the foxglove is used to treat heart disease.

The castor oil plant has been used as a purgative since the time of the Ancient Egyptians.

Cinchona was introduced from Peru in 1492. Its bark contains many alkaloids including quinine.

Sage eases rheumatism and coughs and acts as a disinfectant.

Thyme eases coughs while its oil will act as a sedative and it can also ease toothache.

Ephedrine, a substance which is made from the horsetail plant, was being prescribed as Ma Huang for more than 4,000 years by the Chinese. It is still in use today as an effective relief for asthma.

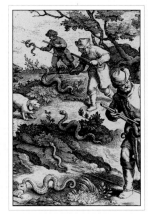

*Theriac was an enormously popular cure-all for six centuries and was often kept in special ornamental jars. Although essentially made from various herbs, a vital ingredient was a powder made from dried vipers – so it could be a profitable enterprise to collect snakes and sell these to apothecaries*

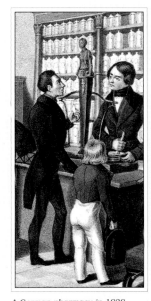

*A German pharmacy in 1838*

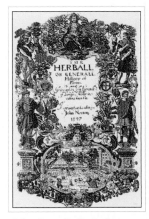

*John Gerard's* Herball, *published in 1597, is still a popular book today*

# ALTERNATIVE

*Left:*

*Ancient medical charts
indicate the 'acupoints' into
which fine needles may be
inserted, according to the
specific treatment*

*Left centre:*

*The Ancient Egyptians
pressed flowers to extract
their juices for medicinal
purposes*

Today there are many alternative approaches to treatment and healing, beyond the confines of conventional medicine as practised by the orthodox practitioner. Many of these are complementary to the treatment offered within the medical profession – but such medication or therapy is best pursued following consultation with a doctor. For many years, medicine in the Western world has been dominated by pharmaceutical drugs and, in recent times, the technology of medicine – but this is now changing and an integrated approach, drawing on both conventional and complementary methods, is becoming acceptable: some doctors have undertaken training in certain complementary therapies in order to be able to offer both kinds of treatment to their patients.

The history of these therapies goes back a very long way. Herbal-based treatments were once the main source of treatment, whilst acupuncture is a very ancient skill, practised in China for thousands of years. Conventional medicine emphasizes a diagnostic approach and focuses on specific problems and symptoms whereas, in general, complementary medicine is more holistic: it treats the whole person and encourages self-healing.

**Here follow a few examples of complementary therapies:**

**Acupuncture**

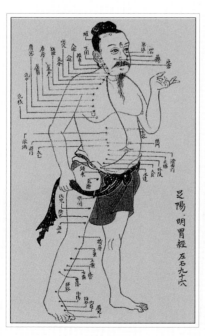

One of the best known Eastern therapies, acupuncture involves inserting fine sterile needles into particular locations on the body. A treatment for disorders and pain relief in the East, generally – in the Western world – it is now accepted as a means of pain relief and anaesthesia.

Ancient stone acupuncture nee-dles found in Inner Mongolia date back to 3,000 BC.

It has been practised widely in China for 2,500 years.

Doctors and missionaries in the 17th century introduced acupuncture into Europe.

The World Health Organisation has named some forty conditions that can be treated with acupuncture.

**Aromatherapy**

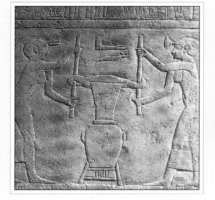

Herbal oils have been used in many cultures throughout history.

Essential oils were used to embalm the dead in Ancient Egypt and recorded by the Ancient Chinese as medicinal. They were also described in the Bible. The oils may be massaged into the body through the skin or inhaled through the nose.

In AD 1000 Persian physician Avicenna developed distillation: the Crusaders introduced his methods into Europe.

In the Middle Ages essential oils were widely used as medicines.

In 1910 French chemist Réné Maurice Gattefossé used lavender oil on his burnt hand and discovered that it healed quickly with little scarring. His studies led to other French doctors, such as Dr Jean Valnet, exploring the use of essential oils.

Essential oils were used to treat wounded soldiers in World War Two.

There has been a recent surge of interest in the effects of aromatherapy and a growing body of practitioners. It is popular as a therapeutic and a useful relaxing technique.

---

**Most commonly
used herbs are:**

Chamomile
Garlic
Ginger
Lavender
Peppermint
Rosemary
Sage
Sandalwood
Tea tree

Clove oil for toothache
Eucalyptus for inhalations

---

**Homeopathy**

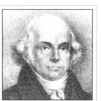

*Samuel
Hahnemann and
his medicine box*

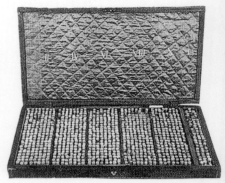

Homeopathy treats the patient as a whole. In 1810, a German doctor, Samuel Hahnemann, founded homeopathy on his therapeutic principle that 'like cures like'. Cinchona produces fever-like symptoms and he therefore argued that what produces fever, also cures fever.

Another completely separate principle of homeopathy is that of 'infinitesimal dosage'. This can be achieved only by vast dilution. This dilution is accompanied by violent shakings – an essential element known as succussion.

Hahnemann's ideas soon spread through Europe, Asia and America. The term homeopathy is derived from the Greek words *homoios* and *pathos* meaning same and suffering, respectively. It remains a popular, but controversial, form of treatment

**Herbalism**

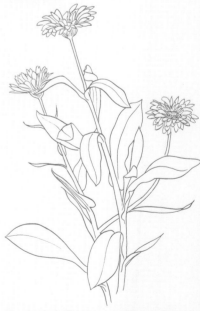

Ancient civilisations in Egypt, Persia, China, India and the Americas were using herbal remedies long before formal European medicine began. Their

use declined a little with the surge of science in the 18th century. Now, however modern clinical research confirms some of the claims made for herbal remedies.

Samuel Thomson set up herbal schools in the USA in the early part of the 19th century.

Modern Western herbalism is now available as a course of study at some universities.

Herbalists claim that the mix of ingredients in plants ('herbal synergy') work as a group – for example, with one chemical perhaps counteracting or alleviating the side effects of another. This provides a more natural balance of chemicals than extracting and isolating, or synthesizing, one particular ingredient.

## Hydrotherapy

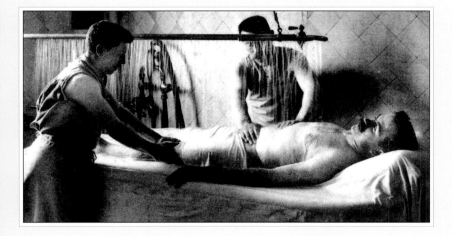

Various uses and forms of water, especially natural hot springs, have been regarded as potential cures for ailments throughout recorded history all around the world.

In Greece, temples to Asklepios, the god of medicine, were mainly raised near hot springs.

The Romans built complexes of baths for immersion in various temperatures.

During the nineteenth century visiting spas to 'take the waters' became very fashionable: the water could be taken both internally or externally.

Father Sebastian Kneipp (1821 1897) was a Bavarian monk who founded modern hydrotherapy. Treatments included hot and cold baths, compresses, foot baths, sitz baths, steam baths, showers, and wraps. (A sitz bath is when the patient sits up to the waist in a hip bath with the feet in another, one hip bath containing hot water, and one cold. The patient keeps changing ends!)

Water alters the blood flow – cold water being stimulating and hot water relaxing – and both hot and cold water have a range of effects on the body systems that can be soothing and/or beneficial.

Steam baths and saunas induce sweating which is believed to elimi-nate impurities from the body.

Today aerated whirlpools, underwater massage and exercise in water are also used as therapy.

## Hypnosis

A state of consciousness between sleep and wakefulness can be induced by a therapist using hypnosis who may then work with patients in this state to causes physical or mental change.

Many ancient texts and tribal traditions include references to inducing trance-like states – with rhythmic dancing and drumming often being used to help achieve this.

Austrian doctor, Franz Mesmer (1734-1815) investigated the powers of 'animal magnetism' and, through this research, began to use powers of suggestion to put patients into a trance and try to bring about cures. Whether or not he was a charlatan, the term 'mesmerise' remains!

Scottish surgeon James Braid (1798-1860) induced hypnotic trances in patients in 1843 and coined the term hypnosis from the Greek word *hypnos* for sleep.

James Esdaile (1808-1859) performed operations in Calcutta using hypnosis for anaesthesia.

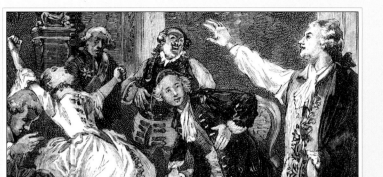

Modern hypnotherapy is now accepted as a complementary therapy. However, no formal training in this area is given to medical students.

## Massage

Massage can be used to treat a countless number of disorders. As well as being soothing and relaxing, it can relieve pain, boost circulation, improve lymphatic and digestive disorders and tone up the muscles.

There are many different techniques and the art of massage goes back to the most ancient civilisations in Egypt, China and India.

In Ancient Greece Hippocrates recommended 'rubbing . . . to bind a joint that is loose, and to loosen a joint that is rigid'.

Later, in Roman times, Julius Caesar had a daily massage to relieve the pain of neuralgia.

Physiotherapy was developed by Swedish gymnast, Per Henrik Ling, and was formally established in the UK in 1894 with the foundation of the Society of Trained Masseurs.

The Touch Research Institute in Miami, USA, reports quite dramatic therapeutic effects from massage – such as premature babies gaining forty-seven per cent more weight and astounding drops in the glucose levels of diabetic children.

*In the 18th century the controversial methods of Franz Anton Mesmer astounded onlookers when he induced hypnotic trances in his patients*

*Left:*
*Treatment with spa water – so popular in Roman times – enjoyed a huge revival in the 19th century*

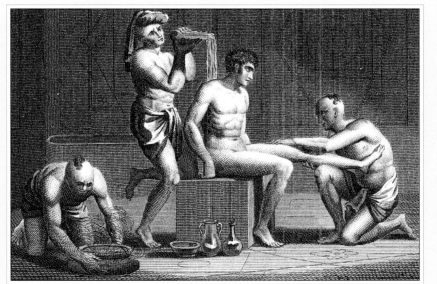

*The benefits of massage have been appreciated throughout medical history*

## Osteopathy

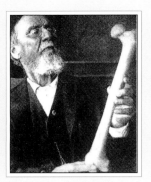

*Osteopathy was 'invented' by Dr Andrew Taylor Still in the USA in 1874. He claimed that, 'all illnesses were due to malpositions of the spine and curable by manipulation'. Modern osteopaths have become more reasonable in their claims and concentrate on their technique of manipulative skills*

Osteopathy is widely practised throughout America, Europe, Japan and Australasia. This is now an established and respected therapy that seeks to relieve problems in the muscular-skeletal system through the means of touch, massage and manipulation. Osteopathy aims to stimulate the body's own natural healing powers and to restore the balance of the body's framework; it is particularly relevant in the treatment of back pain, neck pain and sports injuries but may also be used to relieve arthritis, headaches and insomnia. The name derives from the Greek words for bone *(osteon)* and suffering *(pathos)*.

It was an army doctor from Virginia, Doctor Andrew Taylor Still, who founded the American School of Osteopathy in 1892.

Dr John Martin Littlejohn founded the British School of Osteopathy in 1917.

Dr William Garner developed cranial osteopathy during the 1930s.

Osteopaths have been licensed as doctors in the USA since 1972.

In the UK the Osteopath Act of 1993 granted osteopaths official recognition.

## Reflexology

Reflexology involves massaging specific areas of the foot that are believed to connect in some way to particular organs or parts of the body. Practitioners believe this allows energy channels to flow freely so that damaged areas heal better.

Internal organs and stress-related disorders are the most likely to respond well to reflexology treatment.

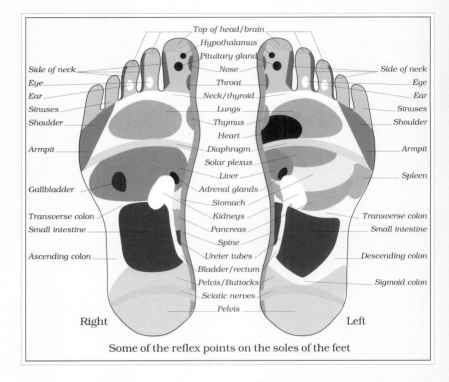

Some of the reflex points on the soles of the feet

At present, there is little scientific evidence to substantiate these claims but the massage is very relaxing and may well work in ways as yet not understood.

The treatment originated in China 5,000 years ago.

Ancient Egyptian wall paintings show a form of manipulation of the feet being used in 2330 BC.

American Dr William introduced zone therapy into the West in 1913.

An American therapist, Eunice Ingham, wrote books on reflexology in the 1930s, detailing reflex points on the hands and feet.

Doreen Bailey set up a reflexology practice and training courses in Britain in 1960.

There are over 7,000 nerve endings in each foot.

# OTHER THERAPIES

### Acupressure
*Began over 3,000 years ago in China.* Ancient system of massage to encourage 'life energy' to flow through body

### Alexander Technique
*Began 1931* Improving posture and stance to relieve stresses on the body. Anthroposophical medicine began 1913 by Rudolf Steiner: a holistic approach encouraging the sense of self and a balance of mind and body

### Bach flower remedies
*Began 1930s* Using healing powers of plants to keep mind and body in harmony

### Bates method
*Early 20th century* Enhancing eyesight without lenses or surgery

### Biochemic tissue salts
*Began 1870s* Using 12 mineral salts to supplement diet intake

### Bioenergetics
*Began 1970s* Psychotherapy: exercises to release physical tension and so relieve mental traumas and anxieties

### Chiropractic
*Began 1895* Spinal manipulation: used to treat spine, joints and muscles and maintain the health of the central nervous system and organs

### Clinical ecology
*Began 1940s* Identifying and avoiding irritants and allergies in the modern environment

### Cranio-sacral therapy
*Began 1970s* Applying pressure to the cranium and spine to stimulate the membranes

### Feldenkrais Method
*Began 1940s* Manipulation and developing awareness of the body through movement

### Hellerwork
*Began 1970s* Massage, body alignment and release of tension

### Meditation
*Began many thousand of years ago.* Evolved through various major religions, introduced into Europe in 19th century, popularised 1960s. Profound relaxation to treat stress-related problems

### Naturopathy
*Began in ancient times. Revived 1895* Using the power of the body to heal itself

### Megavitamin theory
or Orthomolecular *Began 1970s* Treatment with large doses of vitamins, minerals and amino acids

### Rolfing
*Began 1940s* Pressure and manipulation to bring body into appropriate vertical alignment: Improves breathing and suppleness

### Shiatsu
*Began in Ancient China, reached Japan 1,500 years ago, revived in Japan 19th/20th century.* Massage and stimulation at key points to improve energy flow

### T'ai Chi Ch'uan
*Began in 13th century by Taoist monks* Movement and breathing techniques to promote self-healing

### Tragerwork
*Began 1975* Massage, movement and relaxation techniques to re-integrate the body and mind

### Yoga
*Began 5,000 years ago in India* Gentle exercise, postures and breathing techniques

Music, art, light, sound and colour are all also used in a variety of specialised therapies.

# HOW TO
### USE THIS BOOK

This book provides a unique combination of time chart and conventional book pages to create a highly informative document – one that presents all the minutiae which makes up the backbone of the history of medicine in a way that is both clear and accessible.

## The Timechart

### Gatefolds pages 20-36

Each gatefold opens out so that the events through history can be seen as a continuous flow from one page to another.

### Under the flaps

Under the flaps of the gatefolds, there is additional information on a selection of subjects related to the appropriate period of time.

### Streams

The information in the timechart is separated out into various 'streams':

Society
Public health
Disease
Diagnosis
Treatment
Surgery
Healers and teachers
Related skills and practices
Inventions and discoveries
Mental health
Printing and publishing
World events and inventions

This provides an immediate visual display of the ebb and flow of the various elements of history. For example, the widening stream shows how inventions increased

dramatically in the nineteenth century. The narrow stream shows how little emphasis was placed on care of the mentally ill until recent times. Also, when Gutenberg's invention of moveable type meant that printing swept the Western world, to reflect this, a new stream appears for printing and publications.

Occasionally a fact or piece of information may fall into more than one category. In these cases the relevant information may be repeated or cross-referenced.

### Flags and symbols

In order to facilitate seeing the patterns of history at a glance, flags have been used to denote nations (that is, the nations in which the event occurred or in which the perpetrators were born, working or resident, at the time of the event).

The publishers are aware that these are modern flags and that the boundaries of nations, their nomenclature and the flags themselves have mutated over the years. None the less the use of flags (or appropriate symbols for ancient civilisations) remains the simplest and most easily recognised indicator to denote the nations as we understand them today. For example, the EEC flag has been used to denote Europe at a time long before the EEC existed – during the plague of 1642.

We trust, that for reasons of clarity, this will be deemed acceptable as a useful device, if not historically accurate.

## Terminology

Medicine involves some complicated procedures and where the terms involved may not be familiar to the layman, these have been given a brief explanation. However, if space is limited the following terms may appear without explanation:

*Ectopic (or extra-uterine)*
 Pregnancy that occurs outside the womb
*-ectomy*
 Surgery to remove a part
*Excise*
 To cut out or away
*Histology*
 The science of organic tissues
*Otology*
 The science of treating the ear
*Pandemic*
 Universal, spreading through an entire country, continent or the whole world. (An epidemic is confined to a more limited area.)
*Physiology*
 The science or study of natural systems and functions of living things
*Pathology*
 The science or study of disease
*Resection*
 The operation of cutting or paring away a portion of bone or cartilage
*Sutures*
 Joining the lips of a wound or the severed ends of nerves or tendons by stitching
*WHO*
 World Health Organisation

## Factfinder

In order to help trace information the *Factfinder*

links events and personalities to dates and countries. Thus it acts as a useful summary of events as well as an index to lead the reader to the appropriate date on the chart.

### Special subjects

The Timechart has space for only very brief information on any one subject or event.

In order to compensate for this, certain particular areas of interest have been looked at in more detail:

**Disease** and pestilence
**Pharmacy** an ancient art
**Alternative** and complementary medicine.
**Nobel** prize winners
**Women** their role as doctors

### Countries
a brief selection of events

A section on the individual history of various nations has also been included. Inevitably this will repeat information from the main chart but does act as a useful source for seeing a particular nation's history of medicine at a glance.

### Further information

While it is not within the scope of this book to cover all the subject areas of medical history in depth, the comprehensive **Bibliography** and further reading (which includes Internet information) and the list of **Museums** and institutions should enable readers to discover more detailed information about other fields of medical history.

---

| | | | | | |
|---|---|---|---|---|---|
| This gatefold opens, or folds back, giving continuity from the previous page | The names of the streams are repeated on each page | Here the European flag is used in 1500. It refers to the area as we think of it today | Each stream varies in size to indicate the volume of achievements or changes at that time, However, this does not mean that there is no surgery happening in 1530! | | Information under the flap gives more details on some items in this period |

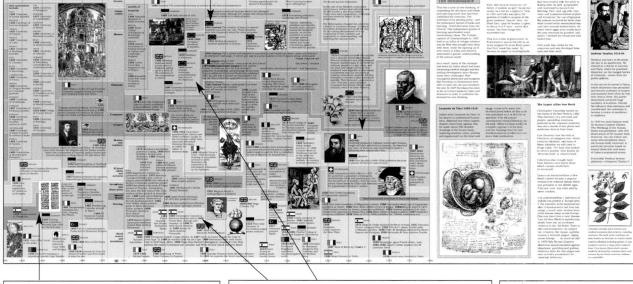

The *Printing and publishing* stream enters the Timechart when Gutenburg invents the first printing press with movable type, thus enabling information to reach more people

*World events and inventions* runs through the Timechart so that the reader can see that, for instance, tropical diseases occur in the West at the same time as Columbus discovers the Americas

To find a specific item in the Timechart refer to the *Fact finder*, page 37, or the *Countries* section, page 62

---

### Facts and figures

Through the course of history, translation from one language into another or misinterpretation have sometimes led to error and confusion. While the publishers have made every effort to verify dates, facts and figures they cannot be held responsible for any misunderstandings, inaccuracies, or controversy! However, they would welcome further information or advice on any such fallible areas – or, indeed, of any advances that occur post-publication – in order to update future editions.

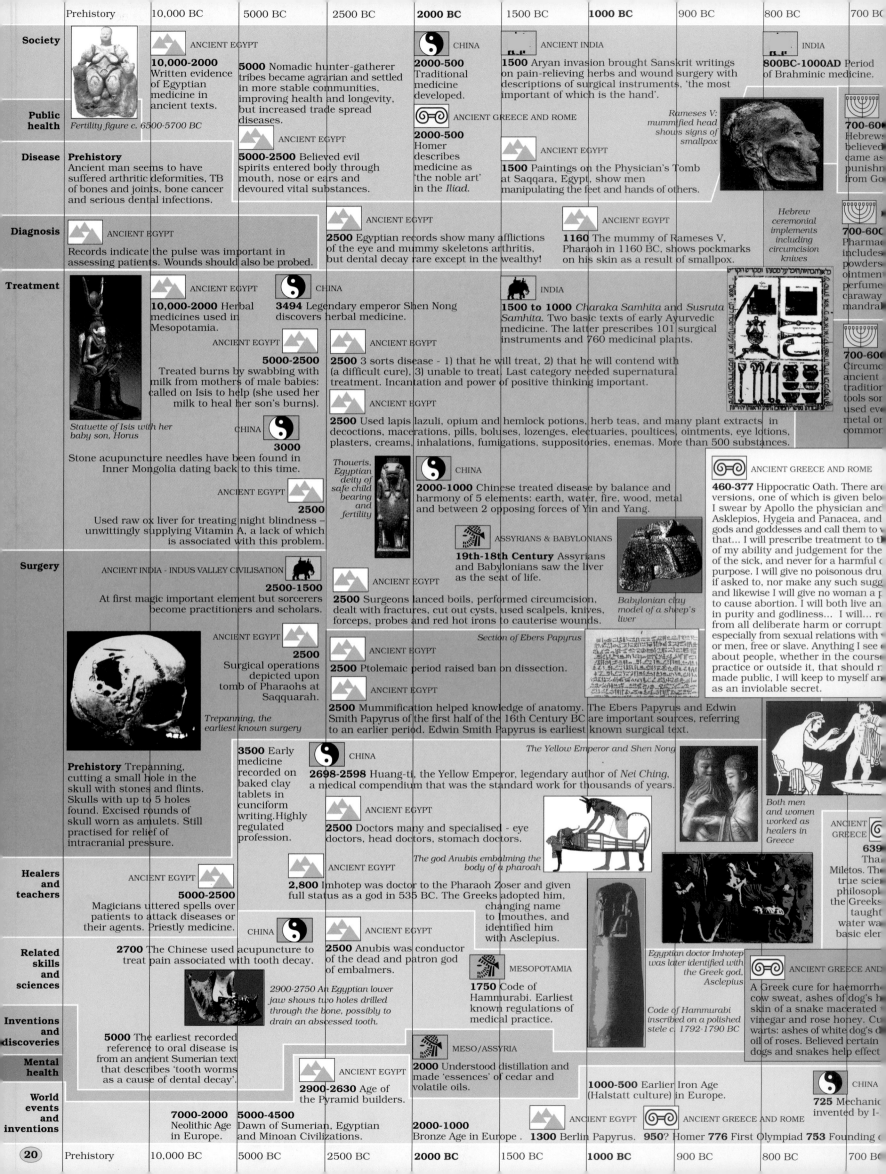

**Society**

ANCIENT EGYPT
**10,000-2000** Written evidence of Egyptian medicine in ancient texts.

*Fertility figure c. 6500-5700 BC*

**5000** Nomadic hunter-gatherer tribes became agrarian and settled in more stable communities, improving health and longevity, but increased trade spread diseases.

CHINA
**2000-500** Traditional medicine developed.

ANCIENT INDIA
**1500** Aryan invasion brought Sanskrit writings on pain-relieving herbs and wound surgery with descriptions of surgical instruments, 'the most important of which is the hand'.

INDIA
**800BC-1000AD** Period of Brahminic medicine.

**Public health**

ANCIENT GREECE AND ROME
**2000-500** Homer describes medicine as 'the noble art' in the *Iliad*.

*Rameses V: mummified head shows signs of smallpox*

**700-60●** Hebrews believed ●came as ●punishm● from Go●

**Disease**

**Prehistory** Ancient man seems to have suffered arthritic deformities, TB of bones and joints, bone cancer and serious dental infections.

ANCIENT EGYPT
**5000-2500** Believed evil spirits entered body through mouth, nose or ears and devoured vital substances.

ANCIENT EGYPT
**1500** Paintings on the Physician's Tomb at Saqqara, Egypt, show men manipulating the feet and hands of others.

**Diagnosis**

ANCIENT EGYPT
Records indicate the pulse was important in assessing patients. Wounds should also be probed.

ANCIENT EGYPT
**2500** Egyptian records show many afflictions of the eye and mummy skeletons arthritis, but dental decay rare except in the wealthy!

ANCIENT EGYPT
**1160** The mummy of Rameses V, Pharaoh in 1160 BC, shows pockmarks on his skin as a result of smallpox.

*Hebrew ceremonial implements including circumcision knives*

**700-600** Pharmac● includes powders ointmen● perfume● caraway● mandrak●

**Treatment**

*Statuette of Isis with her baby son, Horus*

ANCIENT EGYPT
**10,000-2000** Herbal medicines used in Mesopotamia.

CHINA
**3494** Legendary emperor Shen Nong discovers herbal medicine.

ANCIENT EGYPT
**5000-2500** Treated burns by swabbing with milk from mothers of male babies: called on Isis to help (she used her milk to heal her son's burns).

CHINA
**3000** Stone acupuncture needles have been found in Inner Mongolia dating back to this time.

ANCIENT EGYPT
**2500** Used raw ox liver for treating night blindness – unwittingly supplying Vitamin A, a lack of which is associated with this problem.

ANCIENT EGYPT
**2500** 3 sorts disease - 1) that he will treat, 2) that he will contend with (a difficult cure), 3) unable to treat. Last category needed supernatural treatment. Incantation and power of positive thinking important.

ANCIENT EGYPT
**2500** Used lapis lazuli, opium and hemlock potions, herb teas, and many plant extracts in decoctions, macerations, pills, boluses, lozenges, electuaries, poultices, ointments, eye lotions, plasters, creams, inhalations, fumigations, suppositories, enemas. More than 500 substances.

INDIA
**1500 to 1000** *Charaka Samhita* and *Susruta Samhita*. Two basic texts of early Ayurvedic medicine. The latter prescribes 101 surgical instruments and 760 medicinal plants.

**700-600**
Circumc●
ancient
tradition●
tools so●
used eve●
metal or
common

*Thoueris, Egyptian deity of safe child bearing and fertility*

CHINA
**2000-1000** Chinese treated disease by balance and harmony of 5 elements: earth, water, fire, wood, metal and between 2 opposing forces of Yin and Yang.

ASSYRIANS & BABYLONIANS
**19th-18th Century** Assyrians and Babylonians saw the liver as the seat of life.

*Babylonian clay model of a sheep's liver*

ANCIENT EGYPT
**2500** Surgeons lanced boils, performed circumcision, dealt with fractures, cut out cysts, used scalpels, knives, forceps, probes and red hot irons to cauterise wounds.

ANCIENT GREECE AND ROME
**460-377** Hippocratic Oath. There are versions, one of which is given belo● I swear by Apollo the physician and Asklepios, Hygeia and Panacea, and gods and goddesses and call them to ● that... I will prescribe treatment to t● of my ability and judgement for the of the sick, and never for a harmful ● purpose. I will give no poisonous dru● if asked to, nor make any such sugg● and likewise I will give no woman a ● to cause abortion. I will both live an● in purity and godliness... I will... re● from all deliberate harm or corrupt● especially from sexual relations with● or men, free or slave. Anything I see ● about people, whether in the course practice or outside it, that should n● made public, I will keep to myself an● as an inviolable secret.

**Surgery**

*Trepanning, the earliest known surgery*

ANCIENT INDIA - INDUS VALLEY CIVILISATION
**2500-1500** At first magic important element but sorcerers become practitioners and scholars.

ANCIENT EGYPT
**2500** Surgical operations depicted upon tomb of Pharaohs at Saqquarah.

*Section of Ebers Papyrus*

ANCIENT EGYPT
**2500** Ptolemaic period raised ban on dissection.

ANCIENT EGYPT
**2500** Mummification helped knowledge of anatomy. The Ebers Papyrus and Edwin Smith Papyrus of the first half of the 16th Century BC are important sources, referring to an earlier period. Edwin Smith Papyrus is earliest known surgical text.

**Prehistory** Trepanning, cutting a small hole in the skull with stones and flints. Skulls with up to 5 holes found. Excised rounds of skull worn as amulets. Still practised for relief of intracranial pressure.

**3500** Early medicine recorded on baked clay tablets in cunciform writing.Highly regulated profession.

CHINA
**2698-2598** Huang-ti, the Yellow Emperor, legendary author of *Nei Ching*, a medical compendium that was the standard work for thousands of years.

*The Yellow Emperor and Shen Nong*

*Both men and women worked as healers in Greece*

ANCIENT GREECE
**639** Tha● Miletos. The true scien● philosoph● the Greeks taught water wa● basic elem●

**Healers and teachers**

ANCIENT EGYPT
**5000-2500** Magicians uttered spells over patients to attack diseases or their agents. Priestly medicine.

ANCIENT EGYPT
**2500** Doctors many and specialised - eye doctors, head doctors, stomach doctors.

*The god Anubis embalming the body of a pharaoh*

ANCIENT EGYPT
**2,800** Imhotep was doctor to the Pharaoh Zoser and given full status as a god in 535 BC. The Greeks adopted him, changing name to Imouthes, and identified him with Asclepius.

*Egyptian doctor Imhotep was later identified with the Greek god, Asclepius*

**Related skills and sciences**

CHINA
**2700** The Chinese used acupuncture to treat pain associated with tooth decay.

ANCIENT EGYPT
**2500** Anubis was conductor of the dead and patron god of embalmers.

*2900-2750 An Egyptian lower jaw shows two holes drilled through the bone, possibly to drain an abscessed tooth.*

MESOPOTAMIA
**1750** Code of Hammurabi. Earliest known regulations of medical practice.

*Code of Hammurabi inscribed on a polished stele c. 1792-1790 BC*

ANCIENT GREECE AND
A Greek cure for haemorrh● cow sweat, ashes of dog's ● skin of a snake macerated ● vinegar and rose honey. Cu● warts: ashes of white dog's d● oil of roses. Believed certain dogs and snakes help effect

**Inventions and discoveries**

**5000** The earliest recorded reference to oral disease is from an ancient Sumerian text that describes 'tooth worms as a cause of dental decay'.

**Mental health**

ANCIENT EGYPT
**2900-2630** Age of the Pyramid builders.

MESO/ASSYRIA
**2000** Understood distillation and made 'essences' of cedar and volatile oils.

**1000-500** Earlier Iron Age (Halstatt culture) in Europe.

CHINA
**725** Mechanic● invented by I-

**World events and inventions**

**7000-2000** Neolithic Age in Europe.

**5000-4500** Dawn of Sumerian, Egyptian and Minoan Civilizations.

**2000-1000** Bronze Age in Europe .

ANCIENT EGYPT / ANCIENT GREECE AND ROME
**1300** Berlin Papyrus. **950**? Homer **776** First Olympiad **753** Founding of

ANCIENT GREECE AND ROME
**430-427**
Great plague of Athens

ANCIENT GREECE AND ROME
**400**
Thucydides describes Athenian epidemic in his history.

*Asclepius, Greek god of medicine*

INDIA
**500** Ayurvedic medicine can be traced back to 1000 BC but its current form is from this date. They believed the human body is a microcosm of the universe. The body substances (bone, flesh, fat, blood, semen, marrow) are the products of humours: kaph (or phlegm), pitta (or bile), and vata (wind).

*Bas-relief from Barut, India, shows a giant having his tooth extracted*

ANCIENT INDIA
**Century** Surgery extensive inside and outside body. 121 different instruments. Repaired noses with 'plastic surgery', cutting flap from forehead, leaving end over bridge of nose attached. They fixed it in place to nose stump. Wooden tubes inserted to keep artificial 'nostrils' open.

ANCIENT GREECE AND ROME
**3rd Century** Alexandria had 700,000 volumes in library founded by Ptolemy I and a publicly funded research institute in its museum. The library was partly destroyed by fire in 48 BC.

ANCIENT INDIA
**3rd Century** Although not proven, some evidence suggests that Indians may have known malaria came from mosquito and plague carried by rat.

ANCIENT GREECE AND ROME
**234-149** Marcus Porcius Cato, farmer, lawyer, soldier, consul and censor. Collected recipes for medical treatment.

ANCIENT GREECE AND ROME
**370-288** Theophrastus of Eresos. Pupil of Aristotle Author of *Enquiry into Plants*.

ANCIENT GREECE AND ROME
**384-322** Aristotle dissected many species and laid the foundations for embryology. He believed that careful observation, experimentation and the study of cause and effect could lead to greater scientific knowledge.

*Julius Caesar, military genius and shrewd politician, encouraged Roman citizenship and allowed all doctors in Rome to become Roman citizens*

CHINA
**About this time** Deformities of the skeleton were mentioned in Chinese writings of this time. It is not clear whether these abnormalities were the result of rickets.

CHINA
**200** Doctor Zhang Zhongjjing wrote a massive medical book, containing all the medical remedies and treatments known. The book recommends a preparation made from the horsetail plant to ease asthma. The substance is ephedrine, accepted by western doctors in 1923, over 1,700 years after it was first described.

**150 BC** *Attitudes to surgery* Under the Hippocratic oath, using knives and the cutting of patients 'for the stone' had been forbidden to the respected, educated physicians or doctors so surgeons were the less-educated 'craftsmen' who actually undertook these grisly tasks. Later the Church would also strongly oppose dissection and surgery and it was not until the 13th century that the two medical fields were regarded as a whole and equally respected.

ANCIENT GREECE AND ROME
**46** Julius Caesar grants Roman citizenship to all doctors practising in Rome.

ANCIENT GREECE AND ROME
**23** Antonius Musa cures Emperor Augustus of serious illness with his cold water treatment. Doctors granted immunity from taxes.

ANCIENT GREECE AND ROME
**55-63** Lucretius, Roman prefect born 94 BC describes epidemic in *De Rerum Natura*. It contains exposition of doctrines of Epicurus.

ANCIENT GREECE AND ROME
**80** Mithridates VI, King of Pontus 120-63 BC, experiments with poison antidotes. His composition for Theriac contained 41 ingredients.

CHINA
**c 280**
Ts'ang Kung began to study medicine. He wrote 25 case histories - the only records of this kind in Chinese literature for 1,500 years. Described cancer of stomach, cystitis, urinary retention, arthritis, paralysis, aneurysm, haemoptysis and renal disease.

INDIA
**274** The early Indian doctors made house calls. Trained doctors from the Taxila and Barnaras schools worked with physician priests, who combined their skills with religious treatment. In 274 BC hospitals for the care of sick came into existence; the nursing attendants were men.

**The number four**
*The number four assumes an almost magical significance in medical thinking – derived from the balance of the four seasons, the four elements (water, air, fire and earth), the four qualities (moist, dry, hot and cold) and the four humours of the body.*

ANCIENT GREECE AND ROME
**120-70** Asclepiades of Bithynia. Scholars think that almost everything about Asclepiades remains controversial, but he was undoubtedly successful. He held a mechanistic view of the body. Rejected strong drugs in favour of wine, baths and massage. Recommended exercise. Credited in Rome with an ability to arouse the almost dead.

ANCIENT GREECE AND ROME
**120-70** 100 BC
Julius Caesar supposedly delivered by Caesarian section.

ANCIENT GREECE AND ROME
**500-420** Hippocratic school of medicine flourished. Earliest surviving writings of Hippocratic Corpus date from 420 BC.

*Hippocrates*

ANCIENT GREECE AND ROME
**460-377** Hippocrates, leader of medical school and guild in Cos, is regarded as the Father of Western Medicine.

ANCIENT GREECE AND ROME
**280** Herophilus of Chalcedon (330-260). First true anatomist.

ANCIENT GREECE AND ROME
**219**
Arrival of Archagathus, traditionally first Greek doctor to arrive in Rome: was granted Roman citizenship and a public surgery.

ANCIENT GREECE AND ROME
**0-489** Pythagoras founds school Croton. Earliest scientific studies anatomy and physiology.

CHINA
**479-300** *Nei Ching* manual of physic describes acupuncture, originated from work of 2600 BC.

*Already acupuncture had been used in China for many centuries*

ANCIENT GREECE AND ROME
**509** Etruscans pre-Roman. Were skilled dentists and mounted extracted teeth on gold bridges. Gold fillings and dental crowns unearthed.

ANCIENT GREECE AND ROME
**-489**
Alcmaeon Croton discovered optic nerve Eustachian tube of ear.

ANCIENT GREECE AND ROME
**500-428** Anaxagoras believed that each element was composed of many small invisible particles or seeds which were released from food by digestion and then reconstituted into components of the body – such as bone and muscle.

ANCIENT GREECE AND ROME
**200** Just before 200 BC, Archagathus, a Greek Roman citizen, founded first European pharmacy shop near the Forum in Rome. Sold remedies, dressed wounds, had a surgery and hospital.

**The four humours**

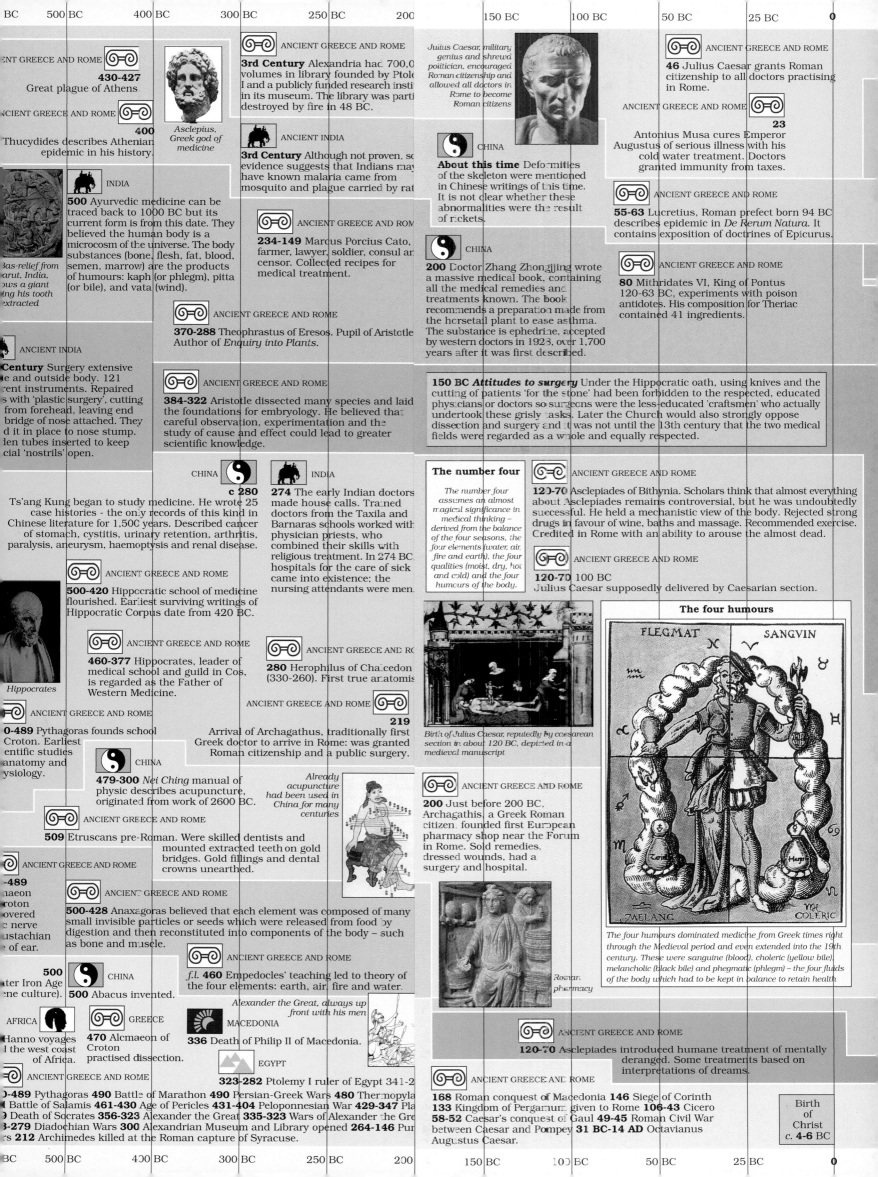

FLEGMAT  SANGVIN
MELANC  COLERIC

*The four humours dominated medicine from Greek times right through the Medieval period and even extended into the 19th century. These were sanguine (blood), choleric (yellow bile), melancholic (black bile) and phegmatic (phlegm) – the four fluids of the body which had to be kept in balance to retain health*

*Birth of Julius Caesar, reputedly by caesarean section in about 120 BC, depicted in a medieval manuscript*

CHINA
**500**
After Iron Age (Shone culture).
**500** Abacus invented.

ANCIENT GREECE AND ROME
*f.l.* **460** Empedocles' teaching led to theory of the four elements: earth, air, fire and water.

*Alexander the Great, always up front with his men*

AFRICA
Hanno voyages the west coast of Africa.

GREECE
**470** Alcmaeon of Croton practised dissection.

MACEDONIA
**336** Death of Philip II of Macedonia.

EGYPT
**323-282** Ptolemy I ruler of Egypt 341-2...

*Roman pharmacy*

ANCIENT GREECE AND ROME
**120-70** Asclepiades introduced humane treatment of mentally deranged. Some treatments based on interpretations of dreams.

ANCIENT GREECE AND ROME

Birth of Christ
*c.* 4-6 BC

## Society

ANCIENT GREECE AND ROME
**69-79** Vespasian frees doctors from military service.

ANCIENT GREECE AND ROME
**200** Medical licensing introduced.

HEBREW
**2-6th Century** The Talmud or book of the law transmitted orally (Mishna) con

## Public health

ANCIENT GREECE AND ROME
**96** Aqueducts carried clean water. (There were sophisticated latrines in forts.) Systems of drains and canals. Controls on conditions of food sales in markets. Orders over burial and cremation, hygiene in public baths.

*Roman toilets, Ephesus*

ANCIENT GREECE AND ROME
c. **397** Fabiola founds first hospital in Western Europe. Eastern hospitals became even larger and more complex.

ANCIENT GREECE AND ROME
Guilds purchased texts and sent them to military forts so medical knowledge spread to every corner of the Roman Empire.

*Hospitals* Ephesus in **420** had with over 75 beds – Jerusalem in had one with 200 beds – St. Sam in Constantinople was even larg Edessa had a women's hospital **400** – Some big hospitals at An and Constantinople were divide **600** into male and female ward

## Disease

ANCIENT GREECE AND ROME
*fl. c.* **98-138** Soranus of Ephesus, Roman founder of obstetrics. His fame rests on his *Diseases of Women*, text used for 15 centuries.

ANCIENT GREECE AND ROME
**357-77** First great Christian hospital at Caesarea founded by Saint Basil.

## Diagnosis

ANCIENT GREECE AND ROME
**79** Plague following eruption of Vesuvius.

ANCIENT GREECE AND ROME
**165-169** Antonine Plague.

ANCIENT GREECE AND ROME
**251-266** Plague of Cyprian.

TURKEY
**541-544** Plague of Justinian. Mediterranean countries.

IRELAND
**675** Monastic r of smallpox in I

## Treatment

ANCIENT GREECE AND ROME
**40-90** Pedanius Dioscorides, a respected army surgeon in time of Nero, writes five-volume *De Materia Medica*, 600 remedies, undisputed authority on plant medicines for over 1,500 years.

ANCIENT GREECE AND ROME
Pharmacy: Theriac, a compound of 61 ingredients including viper meat and opium was a universal antidote. Said to have been invented by Andromarchos c. **54** of Crete, physican to Nero.

ANCIENT GREECE AND ROME
**302** Eusebius, Bishop of Caesarea, describes Syrian epidemic of smallpox.

**541-749** First plague pandemic (spreads to many nations).

*Chinese pulse chart*

CHINA
**280** Wang Shu-ho composed the 12-volume *Mei Ching* (Book of Pulse). Here 'the human body is likened to a chord instrument, of which the different pulses are the chords. The harmony of discord of the organism can be recognised by examining the pulse, which is thus fundamental for all medicine'.

FRANCE
**590** Pandemic of St Anthony's fire (ergotism).

*St Anthony c*

ANCIENT GREECE AND ROM
**600** Aaron, a Christian describes smallpox in h *Pandectae*. This vague ref is cited in the vivid desc of smallpox by Rhazes i *Continens* 860-932.

ANCIENT GREECE AND ROME
**14-37** *De Medicina*, (On Medicine) written by Cornelius Celsus - (8 volumes), who was not a doctor of medicine but knew about clamping veins to prevent haemorrhage, described goitre, cataract, tonsillectomy and plastic surgery. Advised cleaning wounds and defined acute inflammation. We learn an enormous amount about Roman medical thought and practice. Earliest scientific medical work in Latin. Lost for centuries and rediscovered in Siena in 1426.

ANCIENT GREECE AND ROME
**98-117** Rufus of Ephesus wrote on gonorrhoea, anatomy, kidney disease and bedside medicine in *On the interrogation of the patient*.

*Cornelius Celsus*

ANCIENT GREECE AND ROME
**325-403** Oribasius. Provided a treatise on the treatment of fractures by mechanical appliances, including screw traction and elaborate multiple-pulley systems. Composed a medical and surgical encyclopaedia.

FRANCE
**581** Gregory of Tours descri smallpox epidemic at Tours

## Surgery

CHINA
**2nd Century** Warlord Kuan Yun drank wine and played chess while his surgeon, Hua To, cut and scraped out a poisoned arrow wound right down to the bone. When later tried to treat Lord's headache with trepannation Kuan Yun was worried he might have been bribed to murder him and had him executed.

CHINA
**190** Hua To most famous Chinese surgeon who employed anaesthesia using an effervescent powder dissolved in wine. Said to have removed a gangrenous spleen using this method. Surgical advance stopped after his time because of Confucian interdict on mutilation of the human body.

ANCIENT GREECE AND ROME
**357-377** At the first great Christian hospital at Caesarea, the sick, the le the poor and the stranger could receive care and medical assistance. By Edessa, a town of 8,000-10,000 souls, had three small hospitals, supplen in emergencies by beds erected in public colonnades.

ANCIENT GREECE AND ROME
**79** 200 different instruments including vaginal speculum found at Pompeii. Limited anatomical knowledge. →

CHINA
Chinese knowledge of substances to use for treatment is vast and pharmacists handed down knowledge of texts.

CHINA
**6th Century** Castration of eunuchs practised. To reduce pain, a hot decoction of pepper pods applied first to genitals.

CHINA
Precious stones be to have medical p - jade and pearl - ginseng root was considered equa powerful.

## Healers and teachers

*Soranus of Ephesus is regarded as the father of obstetrics*

ANCIENT GREECE AND ROME
**131-201** Galen, born at Pergamum. His first surgical appointment was to the gladiators there. He studied medicine at Alexandria, went to Rome about AD 162 and wrote → extensively on anatomy, physiology and practical medicine, stressing the humoral theory and the Hippocratic doctrine.

ANCIENT GREECE AND ROME
**3rd Century** Martyrdom of Saints Cosmas and Damian. Legend of their grafting a dead Ethiopian's leg on a patient dying of cancer.

ANCIENT GREECE AND ROME
Cupping used by virtually all Roman doctors. A heated bell-shaped metal vessel was placed on the skin to raise a blister and to draw out the 'vicious humour'. Cupping and venesection were also in Arab-Islamic medicine.

ANCIENT GREECE AND
**625-690** Paul of Aeg Discusses tracheoton tonsillectomy, catheterisation, litho and many other surg procedures includin reduction of breast s

ANCIENT GREECE AND ROME
*fl. c.* **98-138** Soranus of Ephesus, first great obstetrician, advised contraception using cotton, ointments or fatty substances. Describes obstetric chair and vaginal speculum, diagnosis of difficulties in labour. Wrote *Signs of Fractures* and *On Acute Chronic Diseases*.

CHINA
*fl.***168-196** Chang Chung-ching was known as the Hippocrates of China. He wrote a classical work on diseases in 16 volumes from a clinical point of view.

ANCIENT GREECE AND ROME    ANCIENT GREECE AND ROME
**502-575**   **525-606** Alexander of Tralles. Skilled phy Aetius of Amida (reign of Justinian I). Masterpiece *Twelve Books on Medicine* Describes ligatures, traumatic aneurysms and diphtheria in his *Tetrabiblon*.

ANCIENT GREECE AND ROME
**158** Galen becomes surgeon to gladiators.

## Related skills and sciences

SWITZERLAND
**570**
Marius, Bishop of Avenches, introduces the term 'variola' (smallpox pustules or pock marks).

FRANCE
Battle of Poitiers 7

## Inventions and discoveries

ANCIENT GREECE AND ROME
**23-79** Pliny the Elder (Caius Plinius Secundus) AD 23-79 great Roman naturalist: his *Natural History* - (37 books) describes drugs obtained from animal, vegetable and mineral sources.

*Pliny and Theophratus*

PLINIVS TEOPHRAST

SPAIN
**711-718**
Conquest of Spain by Muslims

BRITAIN   PERSIA
**450**        **622**
Anglo-Saxons   Mohammed flees conquer      from Mecca to Britain.      Medina (the *Hegira*). Dies in 632.

**642-646** Arab c of Alexandria.

BRI

## Mental health

ANCIENT GREECE AND ROME

**672-735** T Venerable His writing important of history.

## World events and inventions

**c. 30** Christ crucified

**43-57** Roman conquest of Britain **45** Scribonius Largus **54-68** Nero Dioscrides **67-70** Jewish Wars **84** Agricola's Roman fleet circumnavigates Britain **235** Roman civil wars **307-337** Constantine I emperor **330** Foundation of Constantinople as Eastern capital **335** Constantine closes the Asclepieia and other pagan temples. The emperor makes Christianity legal. **360-363** Julian emperor **364** Roman Empire divided **395** Partition of Eastern and Western Roman Empires **410** Goths sack Rome **455** Vandals sack Rome **476** Fall of Western Roman Empire **476** Deposition of Romulus Augustulus, last Western Roman emperor **493-526** Theoderic ruler of Italy.

ANCIENT GREECE AND ROME
**527-565** Justinian emperor.

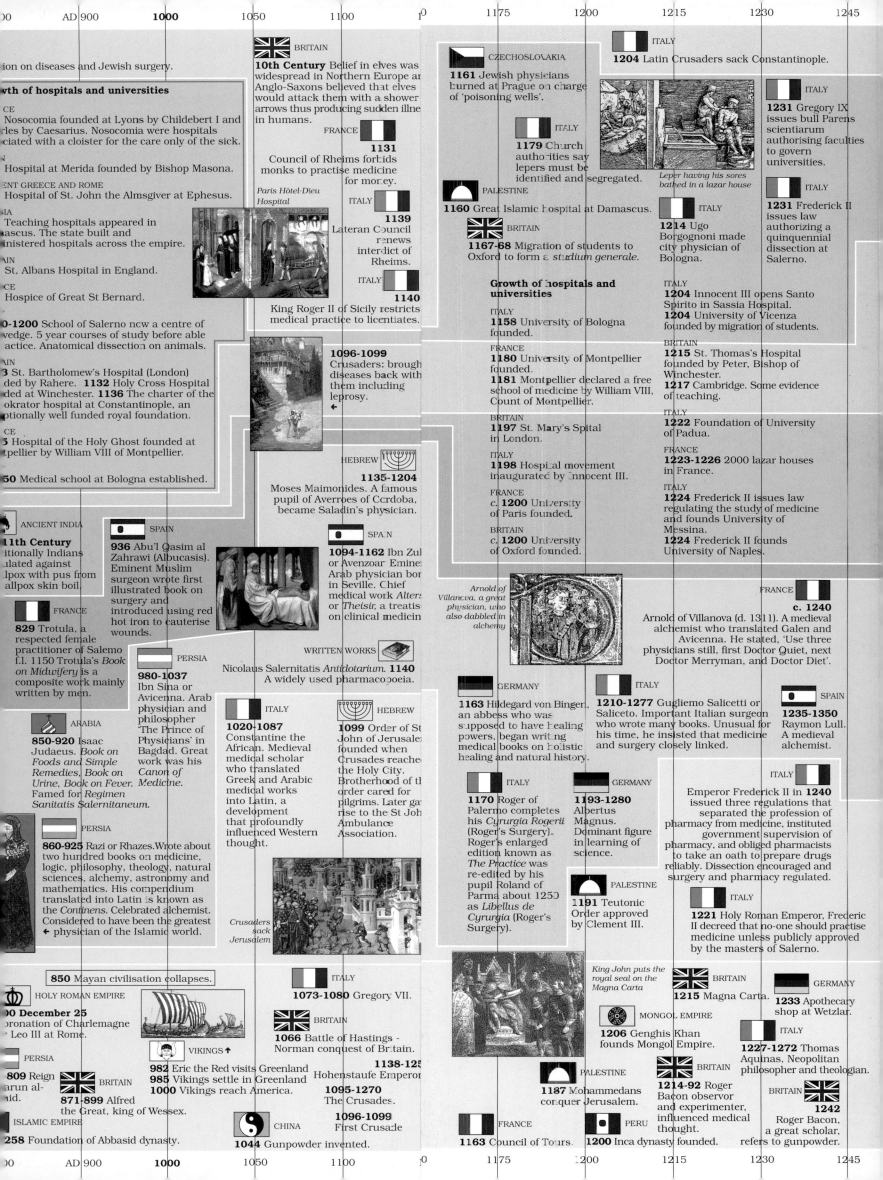

...ion on diseases and Jewish surgery.

**...wth of hospitals and universities**

...CE Nosocomia founded at Lyons by Childebert I and ...rles by Caesarius. Nosocomia were hospitals ...ciated with a cloister for the care only of the sick.

...N Hospital at Merida founded by Bishop Masona.

...ENT GREECE AND ROME Hospital of St. John the Almsgiver at Ephesus.

...SIA Teaching hospitals appeared in ...ascus. The state built and ...inistered hospitals across the empire.

...AIN St. Albans Hospital in England.

...CE Hospice of Great St Bernard.

...0-1200 School of Salerno now a centre of ...wedge. 5 year courses of study before able ...actice. Anatomical dissection on animals.

...AIN 3 St. Bartholomew's Hospital (London) ...ded by Rahere. **1132** Holy Cross Hospital ...ded at Winchester. **1136** The charter of the ...okrator hospital at Constantinople, an ...otionally well funded royal foundation.

...CE 5 Hospital of the Holy Ghost founded at ...tpellier by William VIII of Montpellier.

...50 Medical school at Bologna established.

ANCIENT INDIA
**11th Century** ...itionally Indians ...ulated against ...lpox with pus from ...allpox skin boil.

FRANCE
**829** Trotula, a respected female practitioner of Salerno f.l. 1150 Trotula's *Book on Midwifery* is a composite work mainly written by men.

ARABIA
**850-920** Isaac Judaeus. *Book on Foods and Simple Remedies, Book on Urine, Book on Fever.* Famed for *Regimen Sanitatis Salernitaneum.*

PERSIA
**860-925** Razi or Rhazes. Wrote about two hundred books on medicine, logic, philosophy, theology, natural sciences, alchemy, astronomy and mathematics. His compendium translated into Latin is known as the *Continens.* Celebrated alchemist. Considered to have been the greatest ← physician of the Islamic world.

SPAIN
**936** Abu'l Qasim al Zahrawi (Albucasis). Eminent Muslim surgeon wrote first illustrated book on surgery and introduced using red hot iron to cauterise wounds.

PERSIA
**980-1037** Ibn Sina or Avicenna. Arab physician and philosopher 'The Prince of Physicians' in Bagdad. Great work was his *Canon of Medicine.*

ITALY
**1020-1087** Constantine the African. Medieval medical scholar who translated Greek and Arabic medical works into Latin, a development that profoundly influenced Western thought.

BRITAIN
**10th Century** Belief in elves was widespread in Northern Europe and Anglo-Saxons believed that elves would attack them with a shower ...arrows thus producing sudden illne... in humans.

FRANCE
**1131** Council of Rheims forbids monks to practise medicine for money.

*Paris Hôtel-Dieu Hospital*

ITALY
**1139** Lateran Council renews interdict of Rheims.

ITALY
**1140** King Roger II of Sicily restricts medical practice to licentiates.

**1096-1099** Crusaders: brought diseases back with them including leprosy. ←

HEBREW
**1135-1204** Moses Maimonides. A famous pupil of Averroes of Cordoba, became Saladin's physician.

SPAIN
**1094-1162** Ibn Zul... or Avenzoar. Eminent Arab physician born in Seville. Chief medical work *Alters...* or *Theisir,* a treatise on clinical medicin...

WRITTEN WORKS
Nicolaus Salernitatis *Antidotarium.* **1140** A widely used pharmacopoeia.

HEBREW
**1099** Order of St John of Jerusalem founded when Crusades reached the Holy City. Brotherhood of the order cared for pilgrims. Later gave rise to the St John Ambulance Association.

*Crusaders sack Jerusalem*

CZECHOSLOVAKIA
**1161** Jewish physicians burned at Prague on charge of 'poisoning wells'.

ITALY
**1179** Church authorities say lepers must be identified and segregated.

PALESTINE
**1160** Great Islamic hospital at Damascus.

BRITAIN
**1167-68** Migration of students to Oxford to form a *studium generale.*

**Growth of hospitals and universities**

ITALY
**1158** University of Bologna founded.

FRANCE
**1180** University of Montpellier founded.
**1181** Montpellier declared a free school of medicine by William VIII, Count of Montpellier.

BRITAIN
**1197** St. Mary's Spital in London.

ITALY
**1198** Hospital movement inaugurated by Innocent III.

FRANCE
c. **1200** University of Paris founded.

BRITAIN
c. **1200** University of Oxford founded.

*Arnold of Villanova, a great physician, who also dabbled in alchemy*

GERMANY
**1163** Hildegard von Bingen, an abbess who was supposed to have healing powers, began writing medical books on holistic healing and natural history.

ITALY
**1170** Roger of Palermo completes his *Cyrurgia Rogerii* (Roger's Surgery). Roger's enlarged edition known as *The Practice* was re-edited by his pupil Roland of Parma about 1250 as *Libellus de Cyrurgia* (Roger's Surgery).

GERMANY
**1193-1280** Albertus Magnus. Dominant figure in learning of science.

PALESTINE
**1191** Teutonic Order approved by Clement III.

ITALY
**1204** Latin Crusaders sack Constantinople.

ITALY
**1214** Ugo Borgognoni made city physician of Bologna.

ITALY
**1204** Innocent III opens Santo Spirito in Sassia Hospital.
**1204** University of Vicenza founded by migration of students.

BRITAIN
**1215** St. Thomas's Hospital founded by Peter, Bishop of Winchester.
**1217** Cambridge. Some evidence of teaching.

ITALY
**1222** Foundation of University of Padua.

FRANCE
**1223-1226** 2000 lazar houses in France.

ITALY
**1224** Frederick II issues law regulating the study of medicine and founds University of Messina.
**1224** Frederick II founds University of Naples.

ITALY
**1210-1277** Gugliemo Saliceti or Saliceto. Important Italian surgeon who wrote many books. Unusual for his time, he insisted that medicine and surgery closely linked.

ITALY
**1231** Gregory IX issues bull Parens scientiarum authorising faculties to govern universities.

ITALY
**1231** Frederick II issues law authorizing a quinquennial dissection at Salerno.

*Leper having his sores bathed in a lazar house*

FRANCE
c. **1240** Arnold of Villanova (d. 1311). A medieval alchemist who translated Galen and Avicenna. He stated, 'Use three physicians still, first Doctor Quiet, next Doctor Merryman, and Doctor Diet'.

SPAIN
**1235-1350** Raymon Lull. A medieval alchemist.

ITALY
Emperor Frederick II in **1240** issued three regulations that separated the profession of pharmacy from medicine, instituted government supervision of pharmacy, and obliged pharmacists to take an oath to prepare drugs reliably. Dissection encouraged and surgery and pharmacy regulated.

ITALY
**1221** Holy Roman Emperor, Frederic II decreed that no-one should practise medicine unless publicly approved by the masters of Salerno.

**850** Mayan civilisation collapses.

HOLY ROMAN EMPIRE
...00 December 25 ...ronation of Charlemagne ...y Leo III at Rome.

PERSIA
...809 Reign ...arun al-...id.

BRITAIN
**871-899** Alfred the Great, king of Wessex.

ISLAMIC EMPIRE
...258 Foundation of Abbasid dynasty.

VIKINGS ↑
**982** Eric the Red visits Greenland
**985** Vikings settle in Greenland
**1000** Vikings reach America.

ITALY
**1073-1080** Gregory VII.

BRITAIN
**1066** Battle of Hastings - Norman conquest of Britain.

**1138-125...** Hohenstaufe Emperor...

**1095-1270** The Crusades.

CHINA
**1096-1099** First Crusade
**1044** Gunpowder invented.

*King John puts the royal seal on the Magna Carta*

MONGOL EMPIRE
**1206** Genghis Khan founds Mongol Empire.

PALESTINE
**1187** Mohammedans conquer Jerusalem.

FRANCE
**1163** Council of Tours.

PERU
**1200** Inca dynasty founded.

BRITAIN
**1215** Magna Carta.

GERMANY
**1233** Apothecary shop at Wetzlar.

ITALY
**1227-1272** Thomas Aquinas, Neopolitan philosopher and theologian.

BRITAIN
**1214-92** Roger Bacon observer and experimenter, influenced medical thought.

BRITAIN
**1242** Roger Bacon, a great scholar, refers to gunpowder.

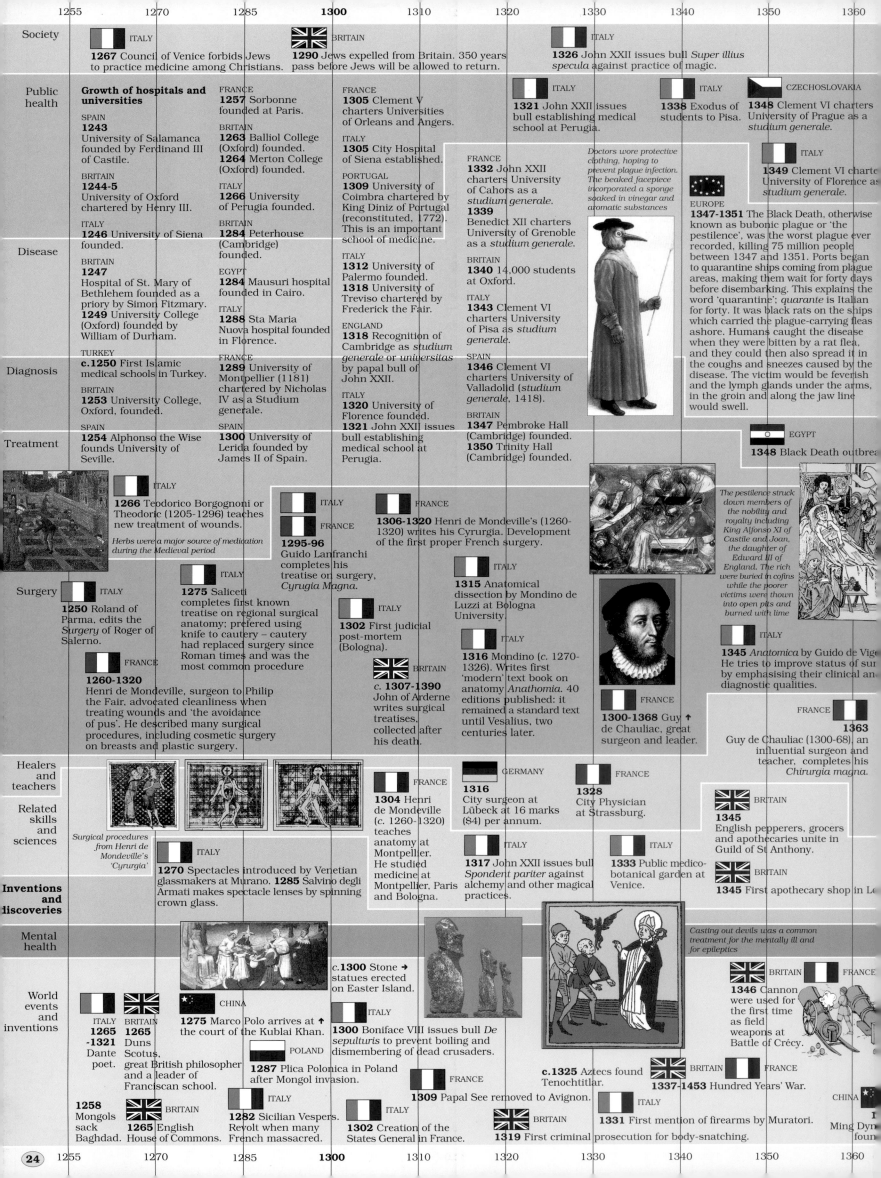

## Society

**ITALY**
**1267** Council of Venice forbids Jews to practice medicine among Christians.

**BRITAIN**
**1290** Jews expelled from Britain. 350 years pass before Jews will be allowed to return.

**ITALY**
**1326** John XXII issues bull *Super illius specula* against practice of magic.

## Public health

**Growth of hospitals and universities**

**SPAIN**
**1243** University of Salamanca founded by Ferdinand III of Castile.

**BRITAIN**
**1244-5** University of Oxford chartered by Henry III.

**ITALY**
**1246** University of Siena founded.

**BRITAIN**
**1247** Hospital of St. Mary of Bethlehem founded as a priory by Simon Fitzmary.
**1249** University College (Oxford) founded by William of Durham.

**FRANCE**
**1257** Sorbonne founded at Paris.

**BRITAIN**
**1263** Balliol College (Oxford) founded.
**1264** Merton College (Oxford) founded.

**ITALY**
**1266** University of Perugia founded.

**BRITAIN**
**1284** Peterhouse (Cambridge) founded.

**EGYPT**
**1284** Mausuri hospital founded in Cairo.

**ITALY**
**1288** Sta Maria Nuova hospital founded in Florence.

**FRANCE**
**1305** Clement V charters Universities of Orleans and Angers.

**ITALY**
**1305** City Hospital of Siena established.

**PORTUGAL**
**1309** University of Coimbra chartered by King Diniz of Portugal (reconstituted, 1772). This is an important school of medicine.

**ITALY**
**1312** University of Palermo founded.
**1318** University of Treviso chartered by Frederick the Fair.

**ENGLAND**
**1318** Recognition of Cambridge as *studium generale* or *universitas* by papal bull of John XXII.

**ITALY**
**1320** University of Florence founded.
**1321** John XXII issues bull establishing medical school at Perugia.

**ITALY**
**1321** John XXII issues bull establishing medical school at Perugia.

**FRANCE**
**1332** John XXII charters University of Cahors as a *studium generale*.
**1339** Benedict XII charters University of Grenoble as a *studium generale*.

**BRITAIN**
**1340** 14,000 students at Oxford.

**ITALY**
**1343** Clement VI charters University of Pisa as *studium generale*.

**SPAIN**
**1346** Clement VI charters University of Valladolid (*studium generale*, 1418).

**BRITAIN**
**1347** Pembroke Hall (Cambridge) founded.
**1350** Trinity Hall (Cambridge) founded.

**ITALY**
**1338** Exodus of students to Pisa.

**CZECHOSLOVAKIA**
**1348** Clement VI charters University of Prague as a *studium generale*.

**ITALY**
**1349** Clement VI charters University of Florence as *studium generale*.

## Disease

*Doctors wore protective clothing, hoping to prevent plague infection. The beaked facepiece incorporated a sponge soaked in vinegar and aromatic substances*

**EUROPE**
**1347-1351** The Black Death, otherwise known as bubonic plague or 'the pestilence', was the worst plague ever recorded, killing 75 million people between 1347 and 1351. Ports began to quarantine ships coming from plague areas, making them wait for forty days before disembarking. This explains the word 'quarantine'; *quarante* is Italian for forty. It was black rats on the ships which carried the plague-carrying fleas ashore. Humans caught the disease when they were bitten by a rat flea, and they could then also spread it in the coughs and sneezes caused by the disease. The victim would be feverish and the lymph glands under the arms, in the groin and along the jaw line would swell.

## Diagnosis

**TURKEY**
**c.1250** First Islamic medical schools in Turkey.

**BRITAIN**
**1253** University College, Oxford, founded.

**SPAIN**
**1254** Alphonso the Wise founds University of Seville.

**FRANCE**
**1289** University of Montpellier (1181) chartered by Nicholas IV as a Studium generale.

**SPAIN**
**1300** University of Lerida founded by James II of Spain.

## Treatment

*Herbs were a major source of medication during the Medieval period*

**ITALY**
**1266** Teodorico Borgognoni or Theodoric (1205-1296) teaches new treatment of wounds.

**EGYPT**
**1348** Black Death outbrea[k]

*The pestilence struck down members of the nobility and royalty including King Alfonso XI of Castile and Joan, the daughter of Edward III of England. The rich were buried in cofins while the poorer victims were thown into open pits and burned with lime*

## Surgery

**ITALY**
**1250** Roland of Parma, edits the *Surgery* of Roger of Salerno.

**FRANCE**
**1260-1320** Henri de Mondeville, surgeon to Philip the Fair, advocated cleanliness when treating wounds and 'the avoidance of pus'. He described many surgical procedures, including cosmetic surgery on breasts and plastic surgery.

**ITALY**
**1275** Saliceti completes first known treatise on regional surgical anatomy; prefered using knife to cautery – cautery had replaced surgery since Roman times and was the most common procedure

**ITALY**
**1295-96** Guido Lanfranchi completes his treatise on surgery, *Cyrugia Magna*.

**ITALY**
**1302** First judicial post-mortem (Bologna).

**FRANCE**
**1306-1320** Henri de Mondeville's (1260-1320) writes his Cyrurgia. Development of the first proper French surgery.

**ITALY**
**1315** Anatomical dissection by Mondino de Luzzi at Bologna University.

**ITALY**
**1316** Mondino (c. 1270-1326). Writes first 'modern' text book on anatomy *Anathomia*. 40 editions published: it remained a standard text until Vesalius, two centuries later.

**BRITAIN**
**c. 1307-1390** John of Arderne writes surgical treatises, collected after his death.

**FRANCE**
**1300-1368** Guy de Chauliac, great surgeon and leader.

**ITALY**
**1345** *Anatomica* by Guido de Vige[vano] He tries to improve status of surg[eons] by emphasising their clinical and diagnostic qualities.

**FRANCE**
**1363** Guy de Chauliac (1300-68), an influential surgeon and teacher, completes his *Chirurgia magna*.

## Healers and teachers
## Related skills and sciences

*Surgical procedures from Henri de Mondeville's 'Cyrurgia'*

**FRANCE**
**1304** Henri de Mondeville (c. 1260-1320) teaches anatomy at Montpellier. He studied medicine at Montpellier, Paris and Bologna.

**GERMANY**
**1316** City surgeon at Lübeck at 16 marks ($4) per annum.

**FRANCE**
**1328** City Physician at Strasbourg.

**BRITAIN**
**1345** English pepperers, grocers and apothecaries unite in Guild of St Anthony.

## Inventions and discoveries

**ITALY**
**1270** Spectacles introduced by Venetian glassmakers at Murano. **1285** Salvino degli Armati makes spectacle lenses by spinning crown glass.

**ITALY**
**1317** John XXII issues bull *Spondent pariter* against alchemy and other magical practices.

**ITALY**
**1333** Public medico-botanical garden at Venice.

**BRITAIN**
**1345** First apothecary shop in Lo[ndon]

## Mental health

*Casting out devils was a common treatment for the mentally ill and for epileptics*

## World events and inventions

**ITALY** **BRITAIN**
**1265 -1321** Dante, poet.
**1265** Duns Scotus, great British philosopher and a leader of Franciscan school.

**1258** Mongols sack Baghdad.

**BRITAIN**
**1265** English House of Commons.

**CHINA**
**1275** Marco Polo arrives at the court of the Kublai Khan.

**POLAND**
**1287** Plica Polonica in Poland after Mongol invasion.

**ITALY**
**1282** Sicilian Vespers. Revolt when many French massacred.

**c.1300** Stone statues erected on Easter Island.

**ITALY**
**1300** Boniface VIII issues bull *De sepulturis* to prevent boiling and dismembering of dead crusaders.

**FRANCE**
**1309** Papal See removed to Avignon.

**ITALY**
**1302** Creation of the States General in France.

**c.1325** Aztecs found Tenochtitlar.

**ITALY**
**1331** First mention of firearms by Muratori.

**BRITAIN**
**1319** First criminal prosecution for body-snatching.

**BRITAIN**
**1337-1453** Hundred Years' War.

**BRITAIN** **FRANCE**
**1346** Cannon were used for the first time as field weapons at Battle of Crécy.

**CHINA**
**[1368]** Ming Dyn[asty] foun[ded]

**BRITAIN**
The Church dominates education and the arts.

**GERMANY**
**1388** Salaried city veterinarian at Ulm.

**ITALY**
**c.1400** Milan institutes permanent health board.

**ITALY**
**1374** Venetian Board of Health/quarantine (*quaranta giorni*) established at Venice in 1403.

Crusaders bought back the Turkish Bath. No fewer than 32 public baths in Paris in 13th Century. However, by 14th Century most baths in England had become brothels.

**EUROPE**
**1377** Ragusa (now Dubrovnic) institutes quarantine.

**EUROPE**
**1400** Epilepsy still seen as an infectious disease. A medical text of the time includes epilepsy in a list of contagious diseases.

**New universities include:**

**USA**
**1474** University of Saragossa.

**ITALY**
**1422** University of Parma founded.

**BELGIUM**
**1426** University of Louvain founded.

**FRANCE**
**1431** University of Poitiers.

**FRANCE**
**1437** University of Caën.

**FRANCE**
**1441** University of Bordeaux founded.

**ITALY**
**1445** University of Catania.

**SPAIN**
**1450** University of Barcelona.

**LUXEMBOURG**
**1450** University of Treves.

**BRITAIN**
**1450** University of Glasgow founded as a *studium generale*.

**GERMANY**
**1456** University of Greifswalds.

**GERMANY**
**1457** University of Freiburg founded.

**GERMANY**
**1459** University of Ingolstadt founded; opened in 1472.

**SWITZERLAND**
**1460** University of Basel founded by citizens of Basel.

**FRANCE**
**1463** University of Nantes.

**FRANCE and HUNGARY**
**1465** Universities at Bourges and Budapest.

**DENMARK**
**1475** University of Copenhagen.

**GERMANY**
**1476** University of Mainz.

**BRITAIN**
**1494** University of Aberdeen founded.

**SPAIN**
**1499** University of Alcala founded.

**SPAIN**
**1501** University of Valencia.

**GERMANY**
**1502** University of Wittenberg constituted as a *studium generale*.

**SPAIN**
**1504** University of Santiago founded.

**SPAIN**
**1505** University of Seville.

**GERMANY**
**1506** University of Frankfurt on the Oder founded.

**SPAIN**
**1508** University of Madrid founded.

**FRANCE**
**1518-1545** Collège de France (Paris).

**SPAIN**
**1526** University of Santiago.

**SPAIN**
**1531** University of Granada.

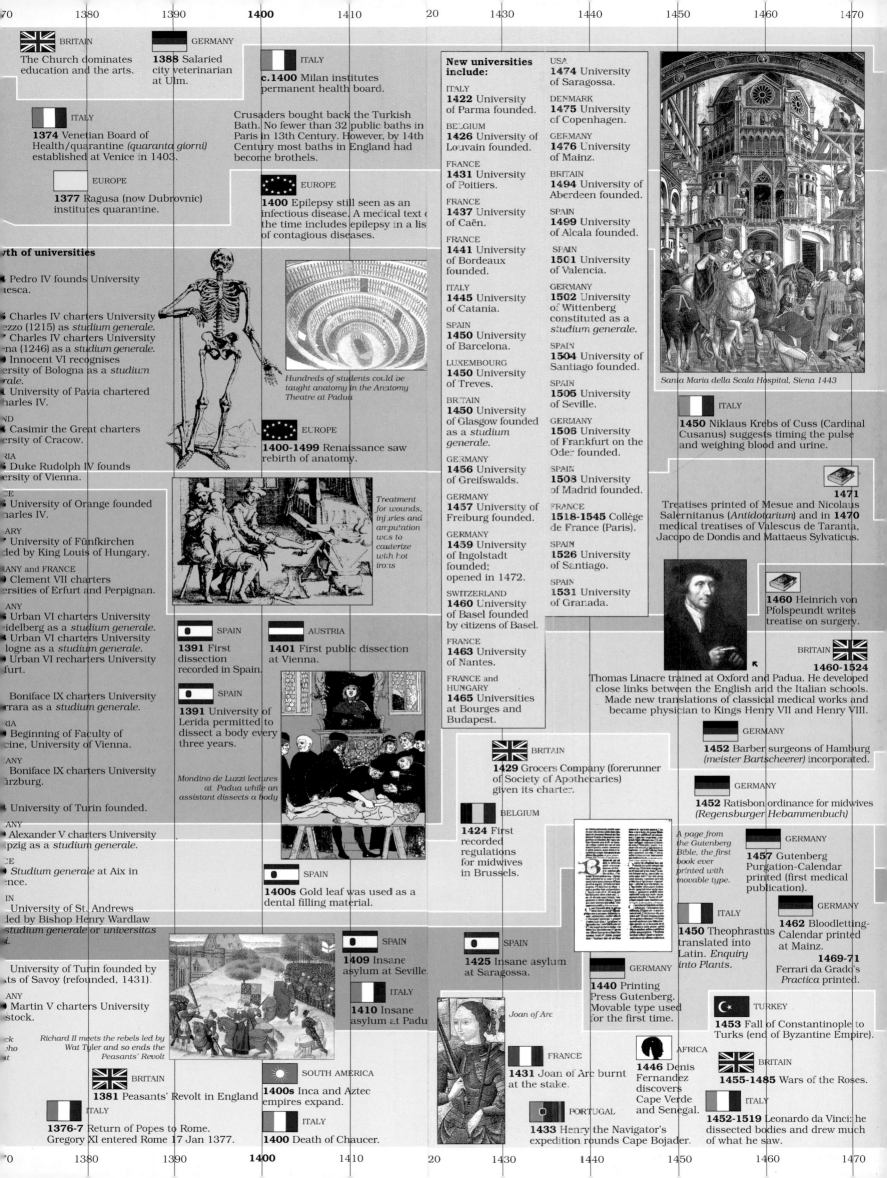

*Santa Maria della Scala Hospital, Siena 1443*

*Hundreds of students could be taught anatomy in the Anatomy Theatre at Padua*

**EUROPE**
**1400-1499** Renaissance saw rebirth of anatomy.

*Treatment for wounds, injuries and amputation was to cauterize with hot irons*

**rth of universities**

Pedro IV founds University esca.

Charles IV charters University ezzo (1215) as *studium generale*.

Charles IV charters University na (1246) as a *studium generale*.

Innocent VI recognises ersity of Bologna as a *studium* ale.

University of Pavia chartered harles IV.

ND Casimir the Great charters ersity of Cracow.

RIA Duke Rudolph IV founds ersity of Vienna.

CE University of Orange founded harles IV.

ARY University of Fünfkirchen ded by King Louis of Hungary.

ANY and FRANCE Clement VII charters ersities of Erfurt and Perpignan.

ANY Urban VI charters University idelberg as a *studium generale*. Urban VI charters University logne as a *studium generale*. Urban VI recharters University furt.

Boniface IX charters University rrara as a *studium generale*.

RIA Beginning of Faculty of cine, University of Vienna.

ANY Boniface IX charters University irzburg.

University of Turin founded.

ANY Alexander V charters University pzig as a *studium generale*.

CE *Studium generale* at Aix in nce.

IN University of St. Andrews ded by Bishop Henry Wardlaw *studium generale* or *universitas* i.

University of Turin founded by ts of Savoy (refounded, 1431).

ANY Martin V charters University stock.

**SPAIN**
**1391** First dissection recorded in Spain.

**SPAIN**
**1391** University of Lerida permitted to dissect a body every three years.

*Mondino de Luzzi lectures at Padua while an assistant dissects a body*

**AUSTRIA**
**1401** First public dissection at Vienna.

**SPAIN**
**1400s** Gold leaf was used as a dental filling material.

**BRITAIN**
**1429** Grocers Company (forerunner of Society of Apothecaries) given its charter.

**BELGIUM**
**1424** First recorded regulations for midwives in Brussels.

**SPAIN**
**1409** Insane asylum at Seville.

**ITALY**
**1410** Insane asylum at Padua.

**SPAIN**
**1425** Insane asylum at Saragossa.

*A page from the Gutenberg Bible, the first book ever printed with movable type.*

**ITALY**
**1450** Theophrastus translated into Latin. *Enquiry into Plants.*

**GERMANY**
**1440** Printing Press Gutenberg. Movable type used for the first time.

*Richard II meets the rebels led by Wat Tyler and so ends the Peasants' Revolt*

**BRITAIN**
**1381** Peasants' Revolt in England

**ITALY**
**1376-7** Return of Popes to Rome. Gregory XI entered Rome 17 Jan 1377.

**SOUTH AMERICA**
**1400s** Inca and Aztec empires expand.

**ITALY**
**1400** Death of Chaucer.

*Joan of Arc*

**FRANCE**
**1431** Joan of Arc burnt at the stake.

**PORTUGAL**
**1433** Henry the Navigator's expedition rounds Cape Bojador.

**AFRICA**
**1446** Denis Fernandez discovers Cape Verde and Senegal.

**ITALY**
**1450** Niklaus Krebs of Cuss (Cardinal Cusanus) suggests timing the pulse and weighing blood and urine.

**1471** Treatises printed of Mesue and Nicolaus Salernitanus (*Antidotarium*) and in **1470** medical treatises of Valescus de Taranta, Jacopo de Dondis and Mattaeus Sylvaticus.

**1460** Heinrich von Pfolspeundt writes treatise on surgery.

**BRITAIN**
**1460-1524** Thomas Linacre trained at Oxford and Padua. He developed close links between the English and the Italian schools. Made new translations of classical medical works and became physician to Kings Henry VII and Henry VIII.

**GERMANY**
**1452** Barber surgeons of Hamburg (*meister Bartscheerer*) incorporated.

**GERMANY**
**1452** Ratisbon ordinance for midwives (*Regensburger Hebammenbuch*)

**GERMANY**
**1457** Gutenberg Purgation-Calendar printed (first medical publication).

**GERMANY**
**1462** Bloodletting-Calendar printed at Mainz.

**1469-71** Ferrari da Grado's *Practica* printed.

**TURKEY**
**1453** Fall of Constantinople to Turks (end of Byzantine Empire).

**BRITAIN**
**1455-1485** Wars of the Roses.

**ITALY**
**1452-1519** Leonardo da Vinci: he dissected bodies and drew much of what he saw.

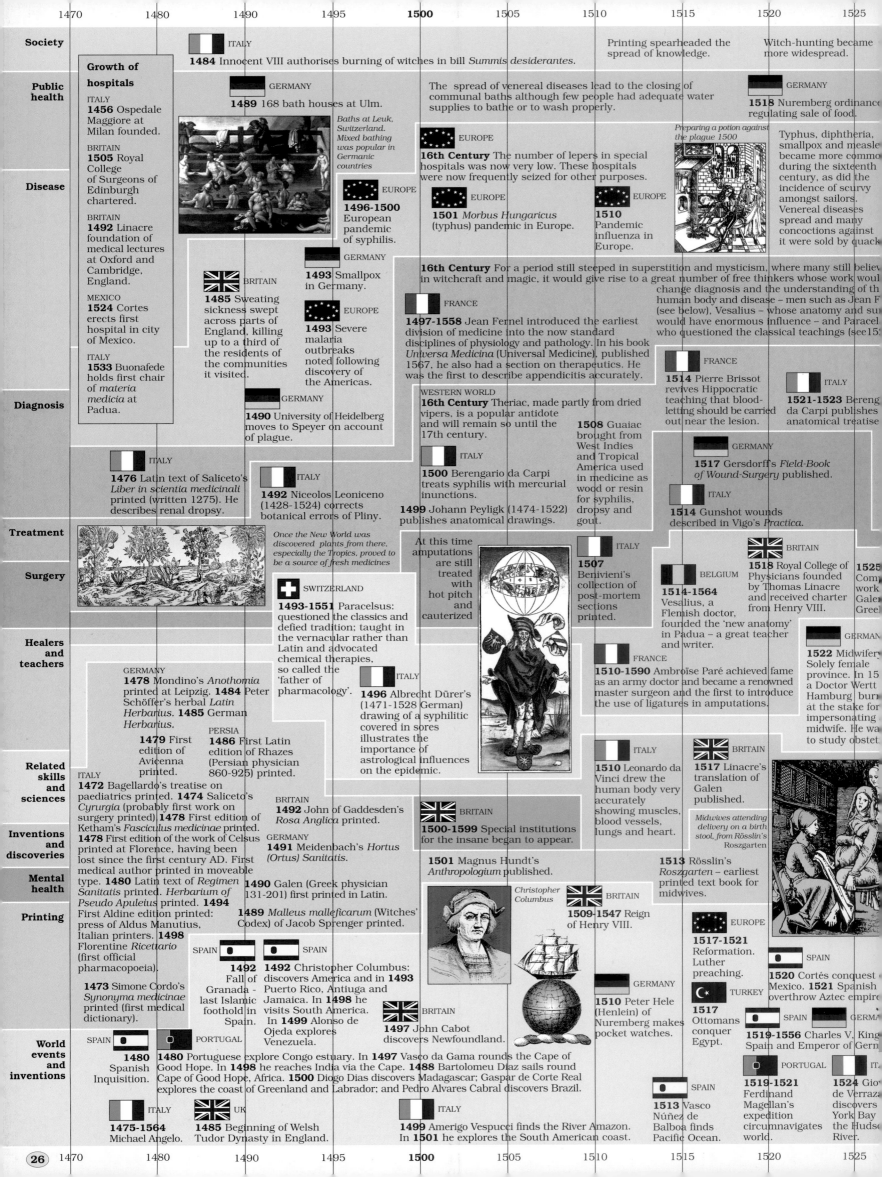

**Society**

ITALY
**1484** Innocent VIII authorises burning of witches in bill *Summis desiderantes*.

Printing spearheaded the spread of knowledge.

Witch-hunting became more widespread.

**Public health**

**Growth of hospitals**

ITALY
**1456** Ospedale Maggiore at Milan founded.

BRITAIN
**1505** Royal College of Surgeons of Edinburgh chartered.

BRITAIN
**1492** Linacre foundation of medical lectures at Oxford and Cambridge, England.

MEXICO
**1524** Cortes erects first hospital in city of Mexico.

ITALY
**1533** Buonafede holds first chair of *materia medicia* at Padua.

GERMANY
**1489** 168 bath houses at Ulm.

The spread of venereal diseases lead to the closing of communal baths although few people had adequate water supplies to bathe or to wash properly.

GERMANY
**1518** Nuremberg ordinance regulating sale of food.

*Baths at Leuk, Switzerland. Mixed bathing was popular in Germanic countries.*

EUROPE
**16th Century** The number of lepers in special hospitals was now very low. These hospitals were now frequently seized for other purposes.

*Preparing a potion against the plague 1500*

Typhus, diphtheria, smallpox and measles became more common during the sixteenth century, as did the incidence of scurvy amongst sailors. Venereal diseases spread and many concoctions against it were sold by quacks.

**Disease**

EUROPE
**1496-1500** European pandemic of syphilis.

EUROPE
**1501** *Morbus Hungaricus* (typhus) pandemic in Europe.

EUROPE
**1510** Pandemic influenza in Europe.

BRITAIN
**1485** Sweating sickness swept across parts of England, killing up to a third of the residents of the communities it visited.

GERMANY
**1493** Smallpox in Germany.

EUROPE
**1493** Severe malaria outbreaks noted following discovery of the Americas.

**Diagnosis**

GERMANY
**1490** University of Heidelberg moves to Speyer on account of plague.

FRANCE
**1497-1558** Jean Fernel introduced the earliest division of medicine into the now standard disciplines of physiology and pathology. In his book *Universa Medicina* (Universal Medicine), published 1567, he also had a section on therapeutics. He was the first to describe appendicitis accurately.

**16th Century** For a period still steeped in superstition and mysticism, where many still believed in witchcraft and magic, it would give rise to a great number of free thinkers whose work would change diagnosis and the understanding of the human body and disease – men such as Jean F[ ] (see below), Vesalius – whose anatomy and su[ ] would have enormous influence – and Paracel[ ] who questioned the classical teachings (see 15[ ]

WESTERN WORLD
**16th Century** Theriac, made partly from dried vipers, is a popular antidote and will remain so until the 17th century.

FRANCE
**1514** Pierre Brissot revives Hippocratic teaching that blood-letting should be carried out near the lesion.

ITALY
**1521-1523** Berengario da Carpi publishes anatomical treatise.

**Treatment**

ITALY
**1476** Latin text of Saliceto's *Liber in scientia medicinali* printed (written 1275). He describes renal dropsy.

ITALY
**1492** Niceolos Leoniceno (1428-1524) corrects botanical errors of Pliny.

ITALY
**1500** Berengario da Carpi treats syphilis with mercurial inunctions.

**1499** Johann Peyligk (1474-1522) publishes anatomical drawings.

**1508** Guaiac brought from West Indies and Tropical America used in medicine as wood or resin for syphilis, dropsy and gout.

GERMANY
**1517** Gersdorff's *Field-Book of Wound-Surgery* published.

ITALY
**1514** Gunshot wounds described in Vigo's *Practica*.

**Surgery**

*Once the New World was discovered plants from there, especially the Tropics, proved to be a source of fresh medicines.*

At this time amputations are still treated with hot pitch and cauterized

ITALY
**1507** Benivieni's collection of post-mortem sections printed.

BELGIUM
**1514-1564** Vesalius, a Flemish doctor, founded the 'new anatomy' in Padua – a great teacher and writer.

BRITAIN
**1518** Royal College of Physicians founded by Thomas Linacre and received charter from Henry VIII.

**1525** Comp[ ] work[ ] Gale[ ] Gree[ ]

**Healers and teachers**

SWITZERLAND
**1493-1551** Paracelsus: questioned the classics and defied tradition; taught in the vernacular rather than Latin and advocated chemical therapies, so called the 'father of pharmacology'.

ITALY
**1496** Albrecht Dürer's (1471-1528 German) drawing of a syphilitic covered in sores illustrates the importance of astrological influences on the epidemic.

FRANCE
**1510-1590** Ambroïse Paré achieved fame as an army doctor and became a renowned master surgeon and the first to introduce the use of ligatures in amputations.

GERMAN[ ]
**1522** Midwifery[ ] Solely female province. In 15[ ] a Doctor Wertt[ ] Hamburg burn[ ] at the stake for impersonating a midwife. He wa[ ] to study obstet[ ]

**Related skills and sciences**

GERMANY
**1478** Mondino's *Anothomia* printed at Leipzig. **1484** Peter Schöffer's herbal *Latin Herbarius*. **1485** German *Herbarius*.

**1479** First edition of Avicenna printed.

PERSIA
**1486** First Latin edition of Rhazes (Persian physician 860-925) printed.

ITALY
**1472** Bagellardo's treatise on paediatrics printed. **1474** Saliceto's *Cyrurgia* (probably first work on surgery printed) **1478** First edition of Ketham's *Fasciculus medicinae* printed. **1478** First edition of the work of Celsus printed at Florence, having been lost since the first century AD. First medical author printed in moveable type. **1480** Latin text of *Regimen Sanitatis* printed. *Herbarium of Pseudo Apuleius* printed. **1494** First Aldine edition printed: press of Aldus Manutius, Italian printers. **1498** Florentine *Ricettario* (first official pharmacopoeia).

BRITAIN
**1492** John of Gaddesden's *Rosa Anglica* printed.

GERMANY
**1491** Meidenbach's *Hortus (Ortus) Sanitatis*.

**1490** Galen (Greek physician 131-201) first printed in Latin.

ITALY
**1510** Leonardo da Vinci drew the human body very accurately showing muscles, blood vessels, lungs and heart.

BRITAIN
**1517** Linacre's translation of Galen published.

*Midwives attending delivery on a birth stool, from Rösslin's Roszgarten*

**Inventions and discoveries**

BRITAIN
**1500-1599** Special institutions for the insane began to appear.

**1501** Magnus Hundt's *Anthropologium* published.

**1513** Rösslin's *Roszgarten* – earliest printed text book for midwives.

**Mental health**

**1473** Simone Cordo's *Synonyma medicinae* printed (first medical dictionary).

**1489** *Malleus malleficarum* (Witches' Codex) of Jacob Sprenger printed.

**Printing**

*Christopher Columbus*

BRITAIN
**1509-1547** Reign of Henry VIII.

EUROPE
**1517-1521** Reformation. Luther preaching.

SPAIN
**1492** Fall of Granada - last Islamic foothold in Spain.

SPAIN
**1492** Christopher Columbus: discovers America and in **1493** Puerto Rico, Antigua and Jamaica. In **1498** he visits South America. In **1499** Alonso de Ojeda explores Venezuela.

GERMANY
**1510** Peter Hele (Henlein) of Nuremberg makes pocket watches.

TURKEY
**1517** Ottomans conquer Egypt.

SPAIN
**1520** Cortés conquest[ ] Mexico. **1521** Spanish overthrow Aztec empire[ ]

**World events and inventions**

SPAIN
**1480** Spanish Inquisition.

PORTUGAL
**1480** Portuguese explore Congo estuary. In **1497** Vasco da Gama rounds the Cape of Good Hope. In **1498** he reaches India via the Cape. **1488** Bartolomeu Diaz sails round Cape of Good Hope, Africa. **1500** Diogo Dias discovers Madagascar; Gaspar de Corte Real explores the coast of Greenland and Labrador; and Pedro Alvares Cabral discovers Brazil.

BRITAIN
**1497** John Cabot discovers Newfoundland.

SPAIN
**1513** Vasco Núñez de Balboa finds Pacific Ocean.

SPAIN
**1519-1556** Charles V, King of Spain and Emperor of Germ[ ]

PORTUGAL
**1519-1521** Ferdinand Magellan's expedition circumnavigates world.

ITALY
**1475-1564** Michael Angelo.

UK
**1485** Beginning of Welsh Tudor Dynasty in England.

ITALY
**1499** Amerigo Vespucci finds the River Amazon. In **1501** he explores the South American coast.

IT[ ]
**1524** Gio[ ] de Verraza[ ] discovers[ ] York Bay[ ] the Hudso[ ] River.

eudal system diminished.

e end of the fifteenth century the
treasury of Rome was collecting some
00 scudos a year from brothels.
e then had a population of 300,000
was served by about 12,000
itutes.

Reformation changed the role of the
ch as countries became Protestant.
deas developed and paved the way
e coming Renaissance with its
ouring of new concepts and
aches to understanding and
ring the natural world.

**ITALY**
**1530** Fracastorius' poem on syphilis published.

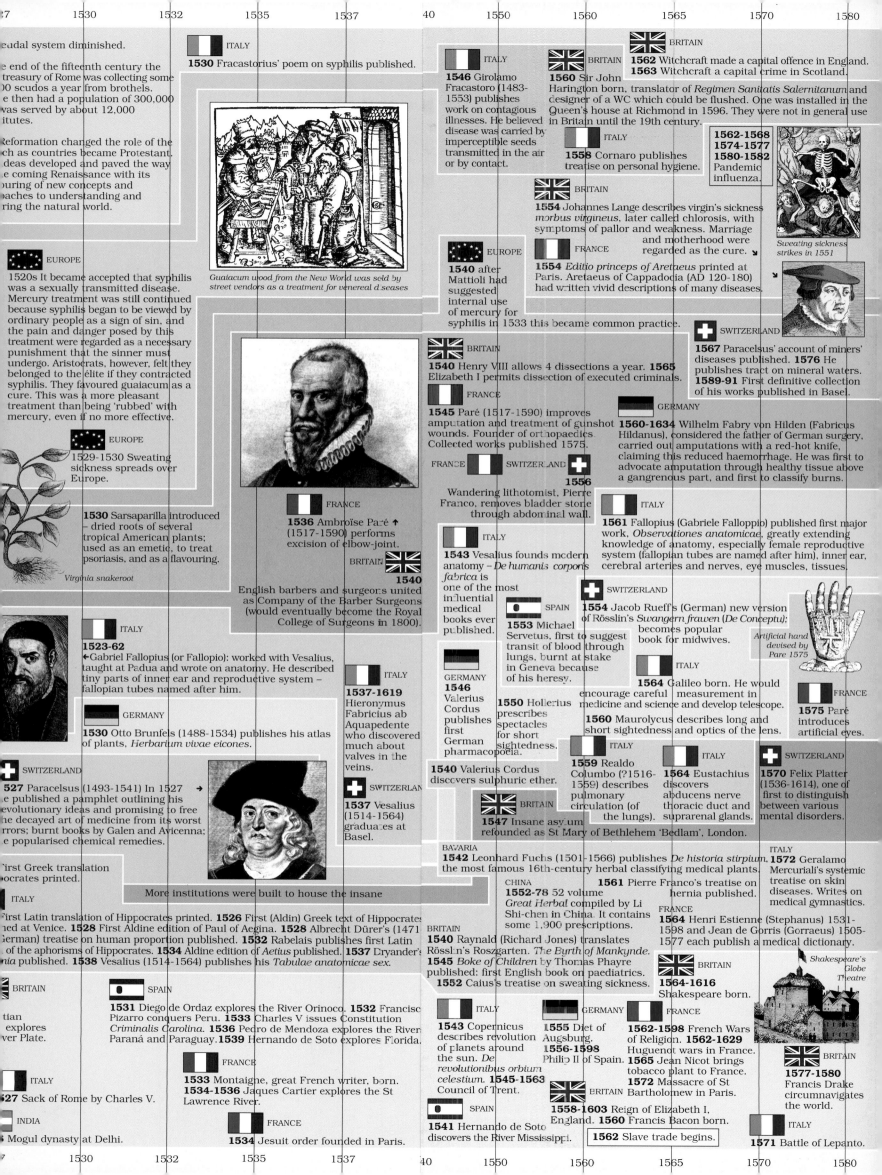
*Guaiacum wood from the New World was sold by street vendors as a treatment for venereal diseases*

**EUROPE**
**1520s** It became accepted that syphilis was a sexually transmitted disease. Mercury treatment was still continued because syphilis began to be viewed by ordinary people as a sign of sin, and the pain and danger posed by this treatment were regarded as a necessary punishment that the sinner must undergo. Aristocrats, however, felt they belonged to the élite if they contracted syphilis. They favoured guaiacum as a cure. This was a more pleasant treatment than being 'rubbed' with mercury, even if no more effective.

**EUROPE**
**1529-1530** Sweating sickness spreads over Europe.

*Virginia snakeroot*

**1530** Sarsaparilla introduced – dried roots of several tropical American plants; used as an emetic, to treat psoriasis, and as a flavouring.

**FRANCE**
**1536** Ambroïse Paré ↑ (1517-1590) performs excision of elbow-joint.

**BRITAIN**
**1540**
English barbers and surgeons united as Company of the Barber Surgeons (would eventually become the Royal College of Surgeons in 1800).

**ITALY**
**1523-62**
←Gabriel Fallopius (or Fallopio): worked with Vesalius, taught at Padua and wrote on anatomy. He described tiny parts of inner ear and reproductive system – fallopian tubes named after him.

**GERMANY**
**1530** Otto Brunfels (1488-1534) publishes his atlas of plants, *Herbarium vivae eicones.*

**SWITZERLAND**
**527** Paracelsus (1493-1541) In 1527
e published a pamphlet outlining his
evolutionary ideas and promising to free
he decayed art of medicine from its worst
rrors; burnt books by Galen and Avicenna;
e popularised chemical remedies.

**ITALY**
**1537-1619** Hieronymus Fabricius ab Aquapedente who discovered much about valves in the veins.

**SWITZERLAND**
**1537** Vesalius (1514-1564) graduates at Basel.

**BAVARIA**
**1542** Leonhard Fuchs (1501-1566) publishes *De historia stirpium,* the most famous 16th-century herbal classifying medical plants.

First Greek translation
ocrates printed.

More institutions were built to house the insane

**ITALY**

First Latin translation of Hippocrates printed. **1526** First (Aldin) Greek text of Hippocrates
ned at Venice. **1528** First Aldine edition of Paul of Aegina. **1528** Albrecht Dürer's (1471-
German) treatise on human proportion published. **1532** Rabelais publishes first Latin
of the aphorisms of Hippocrates. **1534** Aldine edition of *Aetius* published. **1537** Dryander's
nia published. **1538** Vesalius (1514-1564) publishes his *Tabulae anatomicae sex.*

**BRITAIN**

**SPAIN**
**1531** Diego de Ordaz explores the River Orinoco. **1532** Francisco
Pizarro conquers Peru. **1533** Charles V issues Constitution
*Criminalis Carolina.* **1536** Pedro de Mendoza explores the River
Paraná and Paraguay.**1539** Hernando de Soto explores Florida.

tian
explores
ver Plate.

**FRANCE**
**1533** Montaigne, great French writer, born.
**1534-1536** Jaques Cartier explores the St Lawrence River.

**ITALY**
27 Sack of Rome by Charles V.

**INDIA**
Mogul dynasty at Delhi.

**FRANCE**
**1534** Jesuit order founded in Paris.

**ITALY**
**1546** Girolamo Fracastoro (1483-1553) publishes work on contagious illnesses. He believed disease was carried by imperceptible seeds transmitted in the air or by contact.

**BRITAIN**
**1560** Sir John Harington born, translator of *Regimen Sanitatis Salernitanum* and designer of a WC which could be flushed. One was installed in the Queen's house at Richmond in 1596. They were not in general use in Britain until the 19th century.

**BRITAIN**
**1562** Witchcraft made a capital offence in England.
**1563** Witchcraft a capital crime in Scotland.

**ITALY**
**1558** Cornaro publishes treatise on personal hygiene.

**1562-1568
1574-1577
1580-1582** Pandemic influenza.

**BRITAIN**
**1554** Johannes Lange describes virgin's sickness *morbus virgineus,* later called chlorosis, with symptoms of pallor and weakness. Marriage and motherhood were regarded as the cure. ↘

*Sweating sickness strikes in 1551*

**EUROPE**
**1540** after Mattioli had suggested internal use of mercury for syphilis in 1533 this became common practice.

**FRANCE**
**1554** *Editio princeps of Aretaeus* printed at Paris. Aretaeus of Cappadocia (AD 120-180) had written vivid descriptions of many diseases.

**SWITZERLAND**
**1567** Paracelsus' account of miners' diseases published. **1576** He publishes tract on mineral waters. **1589-91** First definitive collection of his works published in Basel.

**BRITAIN**
**1540** Henry VIII allows 4 dissections a year. **1565** Elizabeth I permits dissection of executed criminals.

**FRANCE**
**1545** Paré (1517-1590) improves amputation and treatment of gunshot wounds. Founder of orthopaedics. Collected works published 1575.

**GERMANY**
**1560-1634** Wilhelm Fabry von Hilden (Fabricus Hildanus), considered the father of German surgery, carried out amputations with a red-hot knife, claiming this reduced haemorrhage. He was first to advocate amputation through healthy tissue above a gangrenous part, and first to classify burns.

**FRANCE     SWITZERLAND**
**1556**
Wandering lithotomist, Pierre Franco, removes bladder stone through abdominal wall.

**ITALY**
**1561** Fallopius (Gabriele Falloppio) published first major work, *Observationes anatomicae,* greatly extending knowledge of anatomy, especially female reproductive system (fallopian tubes are named after him), inner ear, cerebral arteries and nerves, eye muscles, tissues.

**ITALY**
**1543** Vesalius founds modern anatomy – *De humanis corporis fabrica* is one of the most influential medical books ever published.

**SPAIN**
**1553** Michael Servetus, first to suggest transit of blood through lungs, burnt at stake in Geneva because of his heresy.

**SWITZERLAND**
**1554** Jacob Rueff's (German) new version of Rösslin's *Swangern frauen (De Conceptu);* becomes popular book for midwives.

*Artificial hand devised by Paré 1575*

**GERMANY**
**1546** Valerius Cordus publishes first German pharmacopoeia.

**1550** Hollerius prescribes spectacles for short sightedness.

**ITALY**
**1564** Galileo born. He would encourage careful measurement in medicine and science and develop telescope.

**1560** Maurolycus describes long and short sightedness and optics of the lens.

**FRANCE**
**1575** Paré introduces artificial eyes.

**1540** Valerius Cordus discovers sulphuric ether.

**BRITAIN**
**1547** Insane asylum refounded as St Mary of Bethlehem 'Bedlam', London.

**ITALY**
**1559** Realdo Columbo (?1516-1559) describes pulmonary circulation (of the lungs).

**ITALY**
**1564** Eustachius discovers abducens nerve thoracic duct and suprarenal glands.

**SWITZERLAND**
**1570** Felix Platter (1536-1614), one of first to distinguish between various mental disorders.

**ITALY**
**1572** Geralamo Mercuriali's systemic treatise on skin diseases. Writes on medical gymnastics.

**CHINA**
**1552-78** 52 volume *Great Herbal* compiled by Li Shi-chen in China. It contains some 1,900 prescriptions.

**1561** Pierre Franco's treatise on hernia published.

**FRANCE**
**1564** Henri Estienne (Stephanus) 1531-1598 and Jean de Gorris (Gorraeus) 1505-1577 each publish a medical dictionary.

**BRITAIN**
**1540** Raynald (Richard Jones) translates Rösslin's Roszgarten. *The Byrth of Mankynde.* **1545** *Boke of Children* by Thomas Phayre published: first English book on paediatrics. **1552** Caius's treatise on sweating sickness.

**BRITAIN**
**1564-1616** Shakespeare born.

*Shakespeare's Globe Theatre*

**ITALY**
**1543** Copernicus describes revolution of planets around the sun. *De revolutionibus orbium celestium.* **1545-1563** Council of Trent.

**GERMANY**
**1555** Diet of Augsburg.
**1556-1598** Philip II of Spain.

**FRANCE**
**1562-1598** French Wars of Religion. **1562-1629** Huguenot wars in France. **1565** Jean Nicot brings tobacco plant to France. **1572** Massacre of St Bartholomew in Paris.

**BRITAIN**
**1558-1603** Reign of Elizabeth I, England. **1560** Francis Bacon born.

**SPAIN**
**1541** Hernando de Soto discovers the River Mississippi.

**1562** Slave trade begins.

**BRITAIN**
**1577-1580** Francis Drake circumnavigates the world.

**ITALY**
**1571** Battle of Lepanto.

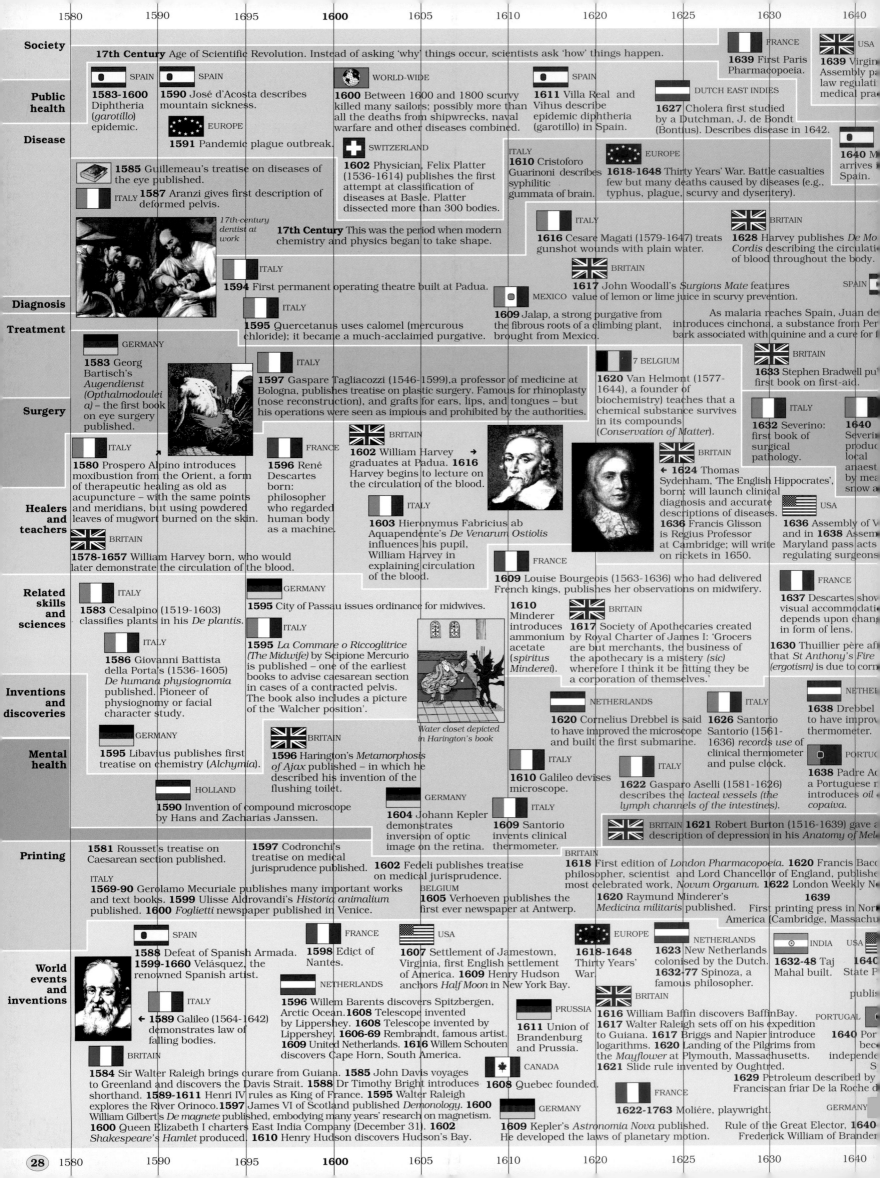

**Society**

**17th Century** Age of Scientific Revolution. Instead of asking 'why' things occur, scientists ask 'how' things happen.

FRANCE **1639** First Paris Pharmacopoeia.

USA **1639** Virginia Assembly passes law regulating medical practice

**Public health**

SPAIN **1583-1600** Diphtheria (*garotillo*) epidemic.

SPAIN **1590** José d'Acosta describes mountain sickness.

WORLD-WIDE **1600** Between 1600 and 1800 scurvy killed many sailors; possibly more than all the deaths from shipwrecks, naval warfare and other diseases combined.

SPAIN **1611** Villa Real and Vihus describe epidemic diphtheria (garotillo) in Spain.

DUTCH EAST INDIES **1627** Cholera first studied by a Dutchman, J. de Bondt (Bontius). Describes disease in 1642.

**Disease**

EUROPE **1591** Pandemic plague outbreak.

**1585** Guillemeau's treatise on the eye published.

ITALY **1587** Aranzi gives first description of deformed pelvis.

SWITZERLAND **1602** Physician, Felix Platter (1536-1614) publishes the first attempt at classification of diseases at Basle. Platter dissected more than 300 bodies.

ITALY **1610** Cristoforo Guarinoni describes syphilitic gummata of brain.

EUROPE **1618-1648** Thirty Years' War. Battle casualties few but many deaths caused by diseases (e.g., typhus, plague, scurvy and dysentery).

SPAIN **1640** M... arrives ... Spain.

*17th-century dentist at work*

**17th Century** This was the period when modern chemistry and physics began to take shape.

ITALY **1616** Cesare Magati (1579-1647) treats gunshot wounds with plain water.

BRITAIN **1628** Harvey publishes *De Mo... Cordis* describing the circulation of blood throughout the body.

**Diagnosis**

ITALY **1594** First permanent operating theatre built at Padua.

BRITAIN **1617** John Woodall's *Surgions Mate* features value of lemon or lime juice in scurvy prevention.

**Treatment**

ITALY **1595** Quercetanus uses calomel (mercurous chloride); it became a much-acclaimed purgative.

MEXICO **1609** Jalap, a strong purgative from the fibrous roots of a climbing plant, brought from Mexico.

As malaria reaches Spain, Juan de ... introduces cinchona, a substance from Per... bark associated with quinine and a cure for ...

**Surgery**

GERMANY **1583** Georg Bartisch's *Augendienst (Opthalmodoulei a)* – the first book on eye surgery published.

ITALY **1597** Gaspare Tagliacozzi (1546-1599),a professor of medicine at Bologna, publishes treatise on plastic surgery. Famous for rhinoplasty (nose reconstruction), and grafts for ears, lips, and tongues – but his operations were seen as impious and prohibited by the authorities.

7 BELGIUM **1620** Van Helmont (1577-1644), a founder of biochemistry) teaches that a chemical substance survives in its compounds (*Conservation of Matter*).

BRITAIN **1633** Stephen Bradwell pu... first book on first-aid.

ITALY **1632** Severino: first book of surgical pathology.

**1640** Severin... produce... local anaest... by mea... snow a...

**Healers and teachers**

ITALY **1580** Prospero Alpino introduces moxibustion from the Orient, a form of therapeutic healing as old as acupuncture – with the same points and meridians, but using powdered leaves of mugwort burned on the skin.

FRANCE **1596** René Descartes born: philosopher who regarded human body as a machine.

BRITAIN **1602** William Harvey graduates at Padua. **1616** Harvey begins to lecture on the circulation of the blood.

ITALY **1603** Hieronymus Fabricius ab Aquapendente's *De Venarum Ostiolis* influences his pupil, William Harvey in explaining circulation of the blood.

**1624** Thomas Sydenham, 'The English Hippocrates', born: will launch clinical diagnosis and accurate descriptions of diseases.

**1636** Francis Glisson is Regius Professor at Cambridge; will write on rickets in 1650.

USA **1636** Assembly of V... and in **1638** Assem... Maryland pass acts regulating surgeons.

BRITAIN **1578-1657** William Harvey born, who would later demonstrate the circulation of the blood.

**Related skills and sciences**

ITALY **1583** Cesalpino (1519-1603) classifies plants in his *De plantis*.

GERMANY **1595** City of Passau issues ordinance for midwives.

FRANCE **1609** Louise Bourgeois (1563-1636) who had delivered French kings, publishes her observations on midwifery.

FRANCE **1637** Descartes show... visual accommodati... depends upon chang... in form of lens.

ITALY **1586** Giovanni Battista della Porta's (1536-1605) *De humana physiognomia* published. Pioneer of physiognomy or facial character study.

ITALY **1595** *La Commare o Riccoglitrice (The Midwife)* by Scipione Mercurio is published – one of the earliest books to advise caesarean section in cases of a contracted pelvis. The book also includes a picture of the 'Walcher position'.

**1610** Minderer introduces ammonium acetate (*spiritus Minderei*).

BRITAIN **1617** Society of Apothecaries created by Royal Charter of James I: 'Grocers are but merchants, the business of the apothecary is a mistery (sic) wherefore I think it be fitting they be a corporation of themselves.'

**1630** Thuillier père affi... that *St Anthony's Fire* (ergotism) is due to corn...

**Inventions and discoveries**

GERMANY **1595** Libavius publishes first treatise on chemistry (*Alchymia*).

BRITAIN **1596** Harington's *Metamorphosis of Ajax* published – in which he described his invention of the flushing toilet.

*Water closet depicted in Harington's book*

NETHERLANDS **1620** Cornelius Drebbel is said to have improved the microscope and built the first submarine.

ITALY **1626** Santorio Santorio (1561-1636) *records use* of clinical thermometer and pulse clock.

NETHER... **1638** Drebbel ... to have improv... thermometer.

**Mental health**

HOLLAND **1590** Invention of compound microscope by Hans and Zacharias Janssen.

ITALY **1610** Galileo devises microscope.

ITALY **1622** Gasparo Aselli (1581-1626) describes the *lacteal vessels (the lymph channels of the intestines)*.

PORTUG... **1638** Padre A... a Portuguese... introduces oil ... copaiva.

GERMANY **1604** Johann Kepler demonstrates inversion of optic image on the retina.

ITALY **1609** Santorio invents clinical thermometer.

BRITAIN **1621** Robert Burton (1516-1639) gave a... description of depression in his *Anatomy of Mel...*

**Printing**

**1581** Rousset's treatise on Caesarean section published.

**1597** Codronchi's treatise on medical jurisprudence published.

ITALY **1569-90** Gerolamo Mecuriale publishes many important works and text books. **1599** Ulisse Aldrovandi's *Historia animalium* published. **1600** *Foglietti* newspaper published in Venice.

**1602** Fedeli publishes treatise on medical jurisprudence.

BELGIUM **1605** Verhoeven publishes the first ever newspaper at Antwerp.

BRITAIN **1618** First edition of *London Pharmacopoeia*. **1620** Francis Baco... philosopher, scientist and Lord Chancellor of England, publishe... most celebrated work, *Novum Organum*. **1622** London Weekly N...

**1620** Raymund Minderer's *Medicina militaris* published.

**1639** First printing press in Nor... America (Cambridge, Massachu...

**World events and inventions**

SPAIN **1588** Defeat of Spanish Armada. **1599-1660** Velásquez, the renowned Spanish artist.

FRANCE **1598** Edict of Nantes.

USA **1607** Settlement of Jamestown, Virginia, first English settlement of America. **1609** Henry Hudson anchors *Half Moon* in New York Bay.

EUROPE **1618-1648** Thirty Years' War.

NETHERLANDS **1623** New Netherland colonised by the Dutch. **1632-77** Spinoza, a famous philosopher.

INDIA **1632-48** Taj Mahal built.

USA **1640** State P... publis...

ITALY **1589** Galileo (1564-1642) demonstrates law of falling bodies.

NETHERLANDS **1596** Willem Barents discovers Spitzbergen, Arctic Ocean. **1608** Telescope invented by Lippershey. **1608** Telescope invented by Lippershey. **1606-69** Rembrandt, famous artist. **1609** United Netherlands. **1616** Willem Schouten discovers Cape Horn, South America.

PRUSSIA **1611** Union of Brandenburg and Prussia.

BRITAIN **1616** William Baffin discovers Baffin Bay. **1617** Walter Raleigh sets off on his expedition to Guiana. **1617** Briggs and Napier introduce logarithms. **1620** Landing of the Pilgrims from the *Mayflower* at Plymouth, Massachusetts. **1621** Slide rule invented by Oughtred.

PORTUGAL **1640** Por... bec... independen...

BRITAIN **1584** Sir Walter Raleigh brings curare from Guiana to Greenland and discovers the Davis Strait. **1588** Dr Timothy Bright introduces shorthand. **1589-1611** Henri IV rules as King of France. **1595** Walter Raleigh explores the River Orinoco. **1597** James VI of Scotland published *Demonology*. **1600** William Gilbert's *De magnete* published, embodying many years' research on magnetism. **1600** Queen Elizabeth I charters East India Company (December 31). **1602** *Shakespeare's Hamlet* produced. **1610** Henry Hudson discovers Hudson's Bay.

CANADA **1608** Quebec founded.

**1629** Petroleum described by Franciscan friar De la Roche d...

FRANCE **1622-1763** Moliére, playwright.

GERMANY **1609** Kepler's *Astronomia Nova* published. He developed the laws of planetary motion.

GERMANY Rule of the Great Elector, **1640**... Frederick William of Brander...

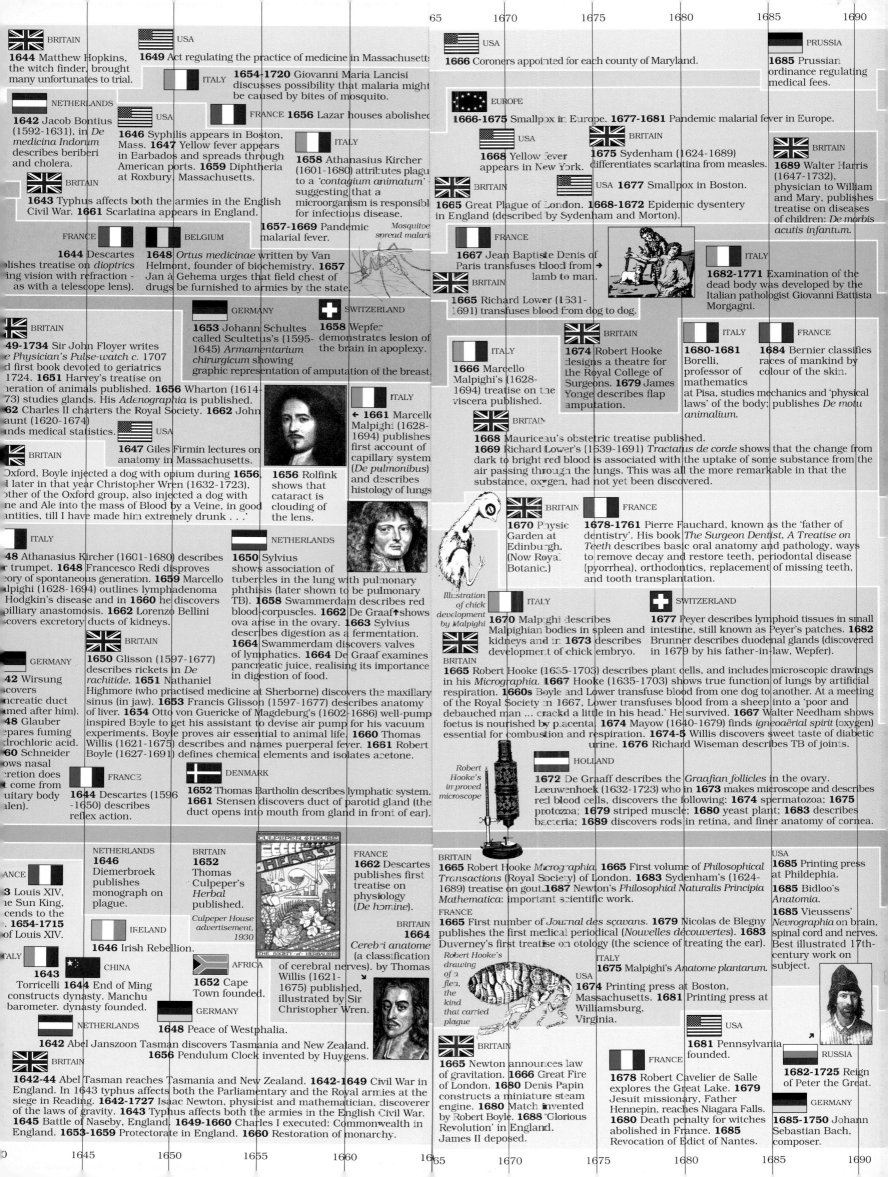

**BRITAIN**
**1644** Matthew Hopkins, the witch finder, brought many unfortunates to trial.

**USA**
**1649** Act regulating the practice of medicine in Massachusetts.

**ITALY**
**1654-1720** Giovanni Maria Lancisi discusses possibility that malaria might be caused by bites of mosquito.

**NETHERLANDS**
**1642** Jacob Bontius (1592-1631), in *De medicina Indorum* describes beriberi and cholera.

**USA**
**1646** Syphilis appears in Boston, Mass. **1647** Yellow fever appears in Barbados and spreads through American ports. **1659** Diphtheria at Roxbury, Massachusetts.

**FRANCE 1656** Lazar houses abolished.

**ITALY**
**1658** Athanasius Kircher (1601-1680) attributes plague to a *'contagium animatum'* suggesting that a microorganism is responsible for infectious disease.

**BRITAIN**
**1643** Typhus affects both the armies in the English Civil War. **1661** Scarlatina appears in England.

**1657-1669** Pandemic malarial fever.

*Mosquitoe spread malaria*

**FRANCE**
**1644** Descartes publishes treatise on *dioptrics* ...ing vision with refraction - as with a telescope lens).

**BELGIUM**
**1648** *Ortus medicinae* written by Van Helmont, founder of biochemistry. **1657** Jan à Gehema urges that field chest of drugs be furnished to armies by the state.

**GERMANY**
**1653** Johann Schultes called Scultetus's (1595-1645) *Armamentarium chirurgicum* showing graphic representation of amputation of the breast.

**SWITZERLAND**
**1658** Wepfer demonstrates lesion of the brain in apoplexy.

**BRITAIN**
**...49-1734** Sir John Floyer writes ...e *Physician's Pulse-watch* c. 1707 ...d first book devoted to geriatrics ...1724. **1651** Harvey's treatise on ...eration of animals published. **1656** Wharton (1614-...73) studies glands. His *Adenographia* is published. **...62** Charles II charters the Royal Society. **1662** John ...aunt (1620-1674) ...nds medical statistics.

**USA**
**1647** Giles Firmin lectures on anatomy in Massachusetts.

**BRITAIN**
...Oxford, Boyle injected a dog with opium during **1656**. ...d later in that year Christopher Wren (1632-1723), ...other of the Oxford group, also injected a dog with ...ne and Ale into the mass of Blood by a Veine, in good ...antities, till I have made him extremely drunk . . .'

**1656** Rolfink shows that cataract is clouding of the lens.

**ITALY**
**...48** Athanasius Kircher (1601-1680) describes ...r trumpet. **1648** Francesco Redi disproves ...ory of spontaneous generation. **1659** Marcello ...lpighi (1628-1694) outlines lymphadenoma ...Hodgkin's disease and in **1660** he discovers ...pillary anastomosis. **1662** Lorenzo Bellini ...covers excretory ducts of kidneys.

**NETHERLANDS**
**1650** Sylvius shows association of tubercles in the lung with pulmonary phthisis (later shown to be pulmonary TB). **1658** Swammerdam describes red blood-corpuscles. **1662** De Graaf shows ova arise in the ovary. **1663** Sylvius describes digestion as a fermentation. **1664** Swammerdam discovers valves of lymphatics. **1664** De Graaf examines pancreatic juice, realising its importance in digestion of food.

**GERMANY**
**...42** Wirsung ...scovers ...ncreatic duct ...amed after him). **...48** Glauber ...epares fuming ...drochloric acid. **...60** Schneider ...ows nasal ...cretion does ...t come from ...uitary body ...alen).

**BRITAIN**
**1650** Glisson (1597-1677) describes rickets in *De rachitide*. **1651** Nathaniel Highmore (who practised medicine at Sherborne) discovers the maxillary sinus (in jaw). **1653** Francis Glisson (1597-1677) describes anatomy of liver. **1654** Otto von Guericke of Magdeburg's (1602-1686) well-pump inspired Boyle to get his assistant to devise air pump for his vacuum experiments. Boyle proves air essential to animal life. **1660** Thomas Willis (1621-1675) describes and names puerperal fever. **1661** Robert Boyle (1627-1691) defines chemical elements and isolates acetone.

**FRANCE**
**1644** Descartes (1596-1650) describes reflex action.

**DENMARK**
**1652** Thomas Bartholin describes lymphatic system. **1661** Stensen discovers duct of parotid gland (the duct opens into mouth from gland in front of ear).

**USA**
**1666** Coroners appointed for each county of Maryland.

**EUROPE**
**1666-1675** Smallpox in Europe. **1677-1681** Pandemic malarial fever in Europe.

**USA**
**1668** Yellow fever appears in New York.

**BRITAIN**
**1675** Sydenham (1624-1689) differentiates scarlatina from measles.

**USA 1677** Smallpox in Boston.

**BRITAIN**
**1665** Great Plague of London. **1668-1672** Epidemic dysentery in England (described by Sydenham and Morton).

**FRANCE**
**1667** Jean Baptiste Denis of Paris transfuses blood from lamb to man.

**BRITAIN**
**1665** Richard Lower (1631-1691) transfuses blood from dog to dog.

**ITALY**
**1666** Marcello Malpighi's (1628-1694) treatise on the viscera published.

**BRITAIN**
**1674** Robert Hooke designs a theatre for the Royal College of Surgeons. **1679** James Yonge describes flap amputation.

**ITALY**
**← 1661** Marcello Malpighi (1628-1694) publishes first account of capillary system (*De pulmonibus*) and describes histology of lungs

**BRITAIN**
**1668** Mauriceau's obstetric treatise published. **1669** Richard Lower's (1639-1691) *Tractatus de corde* shows that the change from dark to bright red blood is associated with the uptake of some substance from the air passing through the lungs. This was all the more remarkable in that the substance, oxygen, had not yet been discovered.

**BRITAIN**
**1670** Physic Garden at Edinburgh. (Now Royal Botanic.)

**FRANCE**
**1678-1761** Pierre Fauchard, known as the 'father of dentistry'. His book *The Surgeon Dentist, A Treatise on Teeth* describes basic oral anatomy and pathology, ways to remove decay and restore teeth, periodontal disease (pyorrhea), orthodontics, replacement of missing teeth, and tooth transplantation.

*Illustration of chick development by Malpighi*

**ITALY**
**1670** Malpighi describes Malpighian bodies in spleen and kidneys and in **1673** describes development of chick embryo.

**SWITZERLAND**
**1677** Peyer describes lymphoid tissues in small intestine, still known as Peyer's patches. **1682** Brunner describes duodenal glands (discovered in 1679 by his father-in-law, Wepfer).

**BRITAIN**
**1665** Robert Hooke (1635-1703) describes plant cells, and includes microscopic drawings in his *Micrographia*. **1667** Hooke (1635-1703) shows true function of lungs by artificial respiration. **1660s** Boyle and Lower transfuse blood from one dog to another. At a meeting of the Royal Society in 1667, Lower transfuses blood from a sheep into a 'poor and debauched man ... cracked a little in his head.' He survived. **1667** Walter Needham shows foetus is nourished by placenta. **1674** Mayow (1640-1679) finds *igneoaërial spirit* (oxygen) essential for combustion and respiration. **1674-5** Willis discovers sweet taste of diabetic urine. **1676** Richard Wiseman describes TB of joints.

*Robert Hooke's improved microscope*

**HOLLAND**
**1672** De Graaff describes the *Graafian follicles* in the ovary. Leeuwenhoek (1632-1723) who in **1673** makes microscope and describes red blood cells, discovers the following: **1674** spermatozoa; **1675** protozoa; **1679** striped muscle; **1680** yeast plant; **1683** describes bacteria; **1689** discovers rods in retina, and finer anatomy of cornea.

**PRUSSIA**
**1685** Prussian ordinance regulating medical fees.

**BRITAIN**
**1689** Walter Harris (1647-1732), physician to William and Mary, publishes treatise on diseases of children: *De morbis acutis infantum*.

**ITALY**
**1682-1771** Examination of the dead body was developed by the Italian pathologist Giovanni Battista Morgagni.

**ITALY**
**1680-1681** Borelli, professor of mathematics at Pisa, studies mechanics and 'physical laws' of the body; publishes *De motu animalium*.

**FRANCE**
**1684** Bernier classifies races of mankind by colour of the skin.

**NETHERLANDS**
**1646** Diemerbroek publishes monograph on plague.

**BRITAIN**
**1652** Thomas Culpeper's *Herbal* published.

*Culpeper House advertisement, 1930*

**FRANCE**
**1662** Descartes publishes first treatise on physiology (*De homine*).

**BRITAIN**
**1664** *Cerebri anatome* (a classification of cerebral nerves), by Thomas Willis (1621-1675) published, illustrated by Sir Christopher Wren.

**BRITAIN**
**1665** Robert Hooke *Micrographia*. **1665** First volume of *Philosophical Transactions* (Royal Society) of London. **1683** Sydenham's (1624-1689) treatise on gout. **1687** Newton's *Philosophial Naturalis Principia Mathematica*: important scientific work.

**FRANCE**
**1665** First number of *Journal des sçavans*. **1679** Nicolas de Blegny publishes the first medical periodical (*Nouvelles découvertes*). **1683** Duverney's first treatise on otology (the science of treating the ear).

**ITALY**
**1675** Malpighi's *Anatome plantarum*.

**USA**
**1674** Printing press at Boston, Massachusetts. **1681** Printing press at Williamsburg, Virginia.

**USA**
**1685** Printing press at Phildephia.
**1685** Bidloo's *Anatomia*.
**1685** Vieussens' *Nevrographia* on brain, spinal cord and nerves. Best illustrated 17th-century work on subject.

**IRELAND**
**1646** Irish Rebellion.

**ITALY**
**1643** Torricelli **1644** constructs barometer.

**CHINA**
**1644** End of Ming dynasty. Manchu dynasty founded.

**AFRICA**
**1652** Cape Town founded.

**NETHERLANDS**
**1642** Abel Janszoon Tasman discovers Tasmania and New Zealand.

**GERMANY**
**1648** Peace of Westphalia.
**1656** Pendulum Clock invented by Huygens.

**FRANCE**
**...3** Louis XIV, ...e Sun King, ...cends to the ...**1654-1715** ...of Louis XIV.

**BRITAIN**
**1642-44** Abel Tasman reaches Tasmania and New Zealand. **1642-1649** Civil War in England. In 1643 typhus affects both the Parliamentary and the Royal armies at the siege in Reading. **1642-1727** Isaac Newton, physicist and mathematician, discoverer of the laws of gravity. **1643** Typhus affects both the armies in the English Civil War. **1645** Battle of Naseby, England. **1649-1660** Charles I executed: Commonwealth in England. **1653-1659** Protectorate in England. **1660** Restoration of monarchy.

**BRITAIN**
**1665** Newton announces law of gravitation. **1666** Great Fire of London. **1680** Denis Papin constructs a miniature steam engine. **1680** Match invented by Robert Boyle. **1688** 'Glorious Revolution' in England. James II deposed.

*Robert Hooke's drawing of a flea, the kind that carried plague*

**FRANCE**
**1678** Robert Cavelier de Salle explores the Great Lake. **1679** Jesuit missionary, Father Hennepin, reaches Niagara Falls. **1680** Death penalty for witches abolished in France. **1685** Revocation of Edict of Nantes.

**USA**
**1681** Pennsylvania founded.

**RUSSIA**
**1682-1725** Reign of Peter the Great.

**GERMANY**
**1685-1750** Johann Sebastian Bach, composer.

## Society

USA **1692** Salem Witchcraft Trials. ↓

FRANCE **1720-1721** Plague in Marseilles.

PRUSSIA **1725** Prussian edict regulating practice of medicine.

BRITAIN 17... English laws agai... witchcraft repeal...

## Public health

**1699** Infectious diseases act in Massachusetts.

*With anatomy now accepted, there was often a shortage of bodies to dissect and body snatching could prove profitable*

EUROPE **1707** Influenza pandemic in Europe.

## Disease

USA **1691** Yellow fever in Boston.

USA **1703-1850** Devastating epidemics of Yellow Fever in tropical and subtropical zones.

BRITAIN **1693-1694** England's Queen Mary II, aged 32, dies of smallpox in a devastating plague that sweeps across Europe.

BRITAIN **1721** Zabdiel Boylston inoculates for smallpox in Boston). **1723** Yellow fever reaches London. **1733** Stephen Hales (1677-1761) *Haemastaticks* describes measurement of blood pressure.

FRANCE **1731** Friedrich Hoffmann (1660-17... describes chlorosis 'Virgin's Disease').

USA Scarlatina appears in the United States **1735**.

## Diagnosis

BRITAIN **1700-1710** Sir John Floyer invents a special pulse watch that runs for exactly one minute.

FRANCE **1705** Brisseau and Maître Jan show that cataract is the clouded lens.

BRITAIN **1714** Daniel Turner (1667-1742): *Treatise of diseases incident to the skin*. Regarded as founder of British dermatology. **1735-1785** John Brown believed that all disease was due to increased excitability (sthenic) or decreased excitability (asthenic). Favourite remedies were laudanum and whisky. The Brunonian system for treating disease involved administrating either sedatives or stimulants.

EUROPE **1729** Influenza pandemic in E... **1732** Another influenza pand... in Europe.

## Treatment

*As watch mechanisms became more accurate so did pulse taking and joined urine examination as a form of clinical diagnosis*

## Surgery

GERMANY **1702** Stahl (1660-1734) states phlogiston theory, concerning combustion and the belief in an invisible 'fire element'.

SWITZERLAND **1736** Haller (1708-1777) points... function of bile in digestion of... Haller was a very important physiolo...

BRITAIN **1726** Stephen Hales (1677-1761) m... first measurement of blood-pressur...

ITALY **1712** Torti of Modena uses ← cinchona bark in pernicious malarial fever.

BRITAIN **1718** Lady Mary Wortley Montagu has son inoculated with smallpox.

BRITAIN **1723** William Cheselden described supra pubic (abdominal wall) surgery for removal of bladder stone.

BRITAIN **1727** Cheselden (1688-1752) performs operation for bladder stones. **1728** Ches... (1688-1752) makes an operation for artificial pupil. **1730** First trache... (incision of windpipe) f... diphtheria by George M...

*A mastectomy operation was performed on this woman by Lorenz Heister in 1720. She did survive*

**1730** Daviel improves cataract operation.

**1736** First succe... operation for appende... by Claudius Ayr...

POLAND **1693** Acoluthus of Breslau resects the lower jaw.

USA **1691** Autopsy of Governor Slaughter in New York.

BRITAIN **1701** Robert Houstoun taps ovarian cyst.

*Prior to anaesthetics, amputees required considerable restraint. Sometimes those who assisted were given the limb as a token*

GERMANY **1716** Surgeon General appointed in German Army at 900 marks per annum. **1718** Heister's (1683-1758) work on surgery published. Lorenz Heister was founder of German scientific surgery.

FRANCE **1721** Palfyn exhibits obstetric forceps to French Academy of Surgery. **1724** Guyot of Versailles attempts catheterisation of the Eustachian tubes in ears.

## Healers and teachers

## Related skills and sciences

BRITAIN **1690** Locke's *Essay on Human Understanding* published.

EUROPE **1692** Jan Cocnan Ammann (1663-1730) teaches deaf-mutes. Methods published in two books, 1692 and 1700.

FRANCE **1713** Dominique Anel catheterises lachrymal (tear) ducts.

SWITZERLAND **1708-1777** Albrecht von Haller, brilliant → writer, botanist and physiologist who studied nervous system.

BRITAIN **1725** John Freind's (1675-1728) *History Physick* published. First English historia... medicine. **1728** John Hunter, scientist, experimenter and surgeon, born.

USA **1730-31** Thomas Cadwalader teaches anatomy in Philadelphi...

GERMANY **1690** Justine Siegemundin publishes treatise on midwifery. **1694** Camerarius gives experimental proof of sexuality in plants.

BRITAIN **1705** Robert Elliot first professor of anatomy at Edinburgh.

FRANCE **1706** First laboratory of marine zoology at Marseilles.

BRITAIN **1724** John Maubray gives private instruction in obstetrics in England. **1726** Chair of midwifery in the University of Edinburgh. Joseph Gibson first Professor of Midwifery in any university. **1726** Edinburgh University appoints a professor of midwifery.

FRANCE **1728** Fauchard (1671-176... publishes *Le chirurgien den...*

*A pharmacy in 1722*

## Inventions and discoveries

BRITAIN **1690** Sir John Floyer counts the pulse by using the watch. **1695** Nehemiah Grew discovers magnesium sulphate in Epsom Waters (Epsom salts). **1730** James Douglas describes the peritoneum. **1733** George Cheyne describes *Cheyne-Stokes respiration*.

GERMANY **1704** Dr Eysenbarth practises as a mountebank in Germany.

BRITAIN **1703** House of Lords authorises apothecaries to prescribe as well as dispense drugs.

USA **1716** New York City issues ordinance for midwives.

NETHERLANDS **1703** Leeuwenhoek (1632-1723) discovers parthenogenesis of plant lice.

ITALY **1710** Santorini's muscle in larynx discovered. **1719** Morgagni (1682-1771) describes syphilis of cerebral arteries.

## Mental health

BRITAIN **1700** Private mad houses were numerous, prosperous and competitive.

ITALY **1700** Ramazzini (1633-1714) publishes treatise on occupational diseases *De morbis artificum diatriba*. **1704** Valsalva (1666-1723) publishes *De aure humana tractatus* and describes *Valsalva's manoeuvre*.

FRANCE **1714** Dominique Anel invents fine point syringe.

GERMANY **1714** Gabriel David Fahrenheit constructs 212 degree mercury thermometer.

BRITAIN **1720** A new theory of consuptions by Benjamin Marten forecasts the existence of the tubercle bacillus.

FRANCE **1730** Réamur (1683-1... introduces 80 degree thermometer.

## Printing and publishing

USA **1693** Printing press in New York.

FRANCE **1700** History and Memoirs of the French Academy of Sciences published.

BRITAIN **1691** Clopton Havers publishes *Osteologia nova* (Haversian canals).

**1707** Dionis' *Cours d'opérations de chirurgie* published.

**1721** Floyer's *Psychrolusia* published.

BRITAIN **1724** Sir John Floyer writes first book devoted to geriatrics.

NETHERLANDS **1732** Boerhaave's *Elementa chemiae* published.

SWED... **1735** Linna... (170... 1778 *Syste... natu... publ...

## World events and inventions

BRITAIN **1698** Steam pump invented by Savery. **1700s** Agricultural Revolution: begins in Britain but then spreads through Europe. **1702-14** Reign of Queen Anne. **1692** Ijsbrand Iders explores the Gobi Desert.

PRUSSIA **1701** Frederick, Elector of Bradenburg, crowned King of Prussia.

RUSSIA **1703** Foundation of St. Petersburg.

*Jethro Tull's seed drill*

FRANCE **1712-78** Philosopher Rousseau born. He will influence French Revolution.

BRITAIN **1712** Steam engine invented by Thomas Newcomen (1663-1729). **1714** Accession of House of Hanover. **1720** Kew Gardens opened.

FRANCE/BRITAIN **1725** A. de Moivre (born in France in 1667, died in Britain in 1754) publishes memoir on *Annuities upon lives*.

FRANCE **1732** Winslow's anatomy published.

DENMARK **1728** Vitus Bering discovers Alaska.

FRANCE **1694-1778** Voltaire.

SPAIN **1701-13** War of the Spanish Succession.

GERMANY **1711** John Shore (George Frederic Handel's trumpeter) invents tuning fork.

SWEDEN Andreas Celsius explores Lapland **1736**.

**GERMANY**
**1740** Friedrich Hoffmann (1660-1742) describes rubella.

**EUROPE**
**1742** Pandemic influenza in Europe.

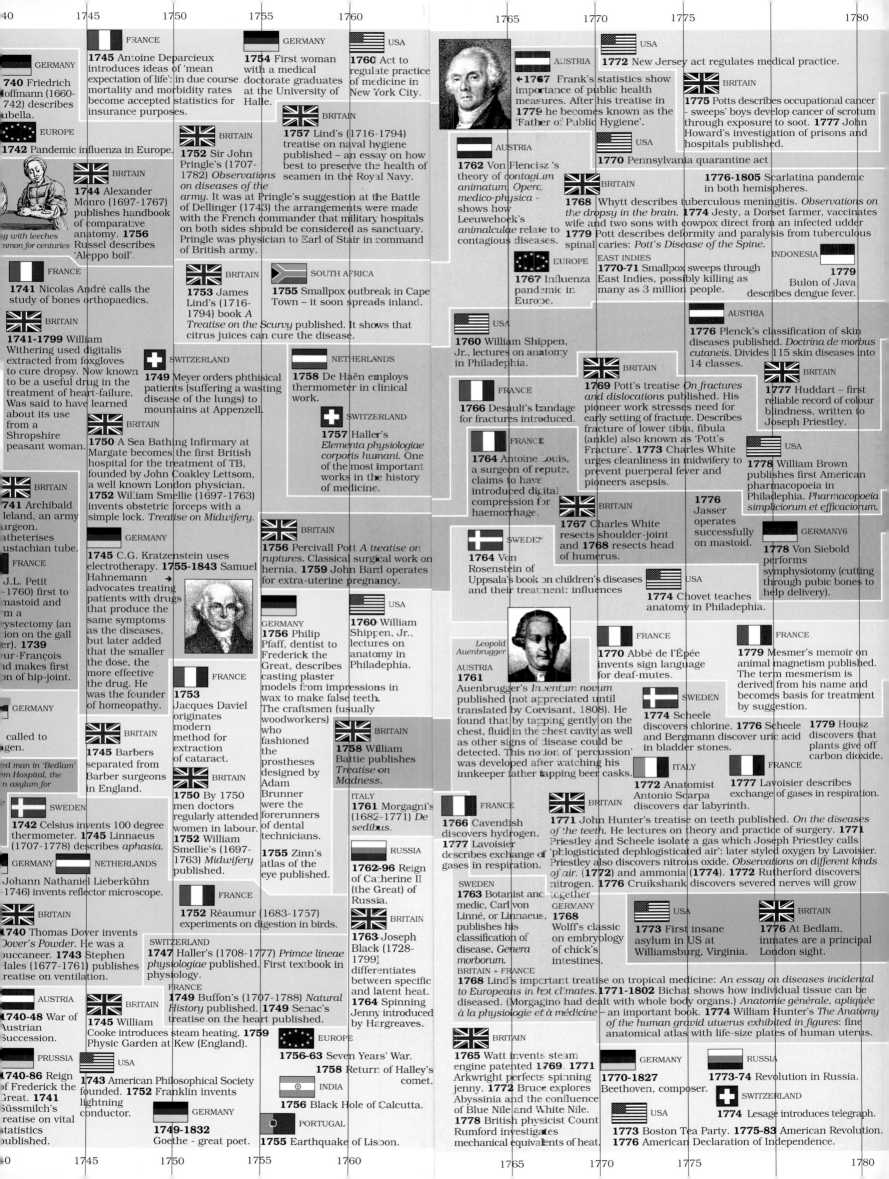

*...g with leeches ...mmon for centuries*

**BRITAIN**
**1744** Alexander Monro (1697-1767) publishes handbook of comparative anatomy. **1756** Russel describes 'Aleppo boil'.

**FRANCE**
**1741** Nicolas André calls the study of bones orthopaedics.

**BRITAIN**
**1741-1799** William Withering used digitalis extracted from foxgloves to cure dropsy. Now known to be a useful drug in the treatment of heart-failure. Was said to have learned about its use from a Shropshire peasant woman.

**BRITAIN**
**1741** Archibald ...leland, an army ...urgeon, ...atheterises ...ustachian tube.

**FRANCE**
J.L. Petit ...-1760) first to ...mastoid and ...m a ...ystectomy (an ...ion on the gall ...er). **1739** ...ur-François ...d makes first ...on of hip-joint.

**GERMANY**
...called to ...gen.

[engraving] *...ed man in 'Bedlam' ...rm Hospital, the ...n asylum for*

**BRITAIN**
**1745** Barbers separated from Barber surgeons in England.

**SWEDEN**
**1742** Celsius invents 100 degree thermometer. **1745** Linnaeus (1707-1778) describes *aphasia*.

**GERMANY** **NETHERLANDS**
Johann Nathaniel Lieberkühn ...-1746) invents reflector microscope.

**BRITAIN**
**1740** Thomas Dover invents *Dover's Powder*. He was a ...buccaneer. **1743** Stephen ...Hales (1677-1761) publishes ...treatise on ventilation.

**AUSTRIA**
**1740-48** War of ...Austrian ...Succession.

**PRUSSIA**
**1740-86** Reign ...of Frederick the ...Great. **1741** ...Süssmilch's ...treatise on vital ...statistics ...published.

**FRANCE**
**1745** Antoine Deparcieux introduces ideas of 'mean expectation of life': in due course mortality and morbidity rates become accepted statistics for insurance purposes.

**BRITAIN**
**1752** Sir John Pringle's (1707-1782) *Observations on diseases of the army*. It was at Pringle's suggestion at the Battle of Dellinger (1743) the arrangements were made with the French commander that military hospitals on both sides should be considered as sanctuary. Pringle was physician to Earl of Stair in command of British army.

**BRITAIN**
**1753** James Lind's (1716-1794) book *A Treatise on the Scurvy* published. It shows that citrus juices can cure the disease.

**SWITZERLAND**
**1749** Meyer orders phthisical patients (suffering a wasting disease of the lungs) to mountains at Appenzell.

**BRITAIN**
**1750** A Sea Bathing Infirmary at Margate becomes the first British hospital for the treatment of TB, founded by John Coakley Lettsom, a well known London physician. **1752** William Smellie (1697-1763) invents obstetric forceps with a simple lock. *Treatise on Midwifery.*

**GERMANY**
**1745** C.G. Kratzenstein uses electrotherapy. **1755-1843** Samuel Hahnemann → advocates treating patients with drugs that produce the same symptoms as the diseases, but later added that the smaller the dose, the more effective the drug. He was the founder of homeopathy.

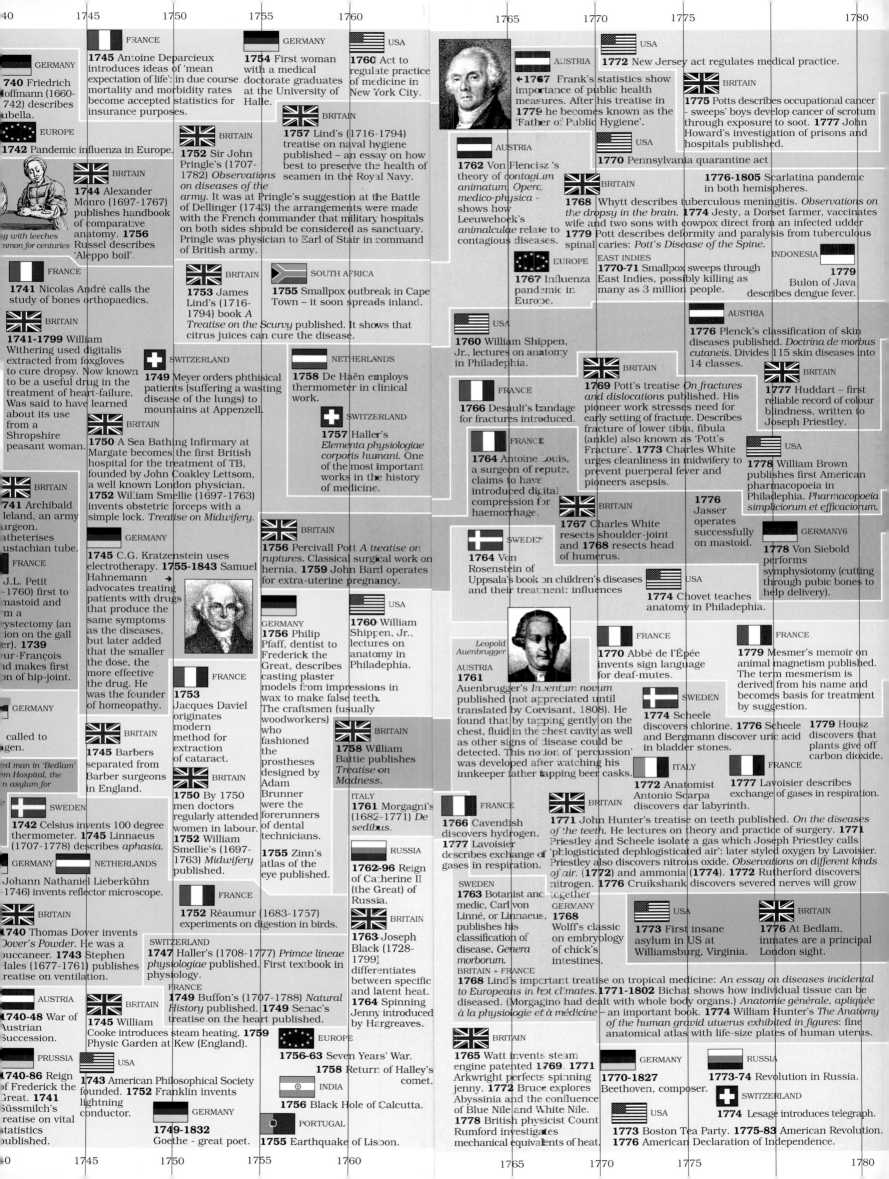

**FRANCE**
**1753** Jacques Daviel originates modern method for extraction of cataract.

**BRITAIN**
**1750** By 1750 men doctors regularly attended women in labour. **1752** William Smellie's (1697-1763) *Midwifery* published.

**FRANCE**
**1752** Réaumur (1683-1757) experiments on digestion in birds.

**SWITZERLAND**
**1747** Haller's (1708-1777) *Primae lineae physiologiae* published. First textbook in physiology.

**FRANCE**
**1749** Buffon's (1707-1788) *Natural History* published. **1749** Senac's treatise on the heart published.

**BRITAIN**
**1745** William Cooke introduces steam heating. **1759** Physic Garden at Kew (England).

**USA**
**1743** American Philosophical Society founded. **1752** Franklin invents lightning conductor.

**GERMANY**
**1749-1832** Goethe - great poet.

**GERMANY**
**1754** First woman with a medical doctorate graduates at the University of Halle.

**BRITAIN**
**1757** Lind's (1716-1794) treatise on naval hygiene published – an essay on how best to preserve the health of seamen in the Royal Navy.

**SOUTH AFRICA**
**1755** Smallpox outbreak in Cape Town – it soon spreads inland.

**NETHERLANDS**
**1758** De Haën employs thermometer in clinical work.

**SWITZERLAND**
**1757** Haller's *Elementa physiologiae corporis humani*. One of the most important works in the history of medicine.

**BRITAIN**
**1756** Percivall Pott *A treatise on ruptures*. Classical surgical work on hernia. **1759** John Bard operates for extra-uterine pregnancy.

**GERMANY**
**1756** Philip Pfaff, dentist to Frederick the Great, describes casting plaster models from impressions in wax to make false teeth. The craftsmen (usually woodworkers) who fashioned the prostheses designed by Adam Brunner were the forerunners of dental technicians.

**BRITAIN**
**1758** William Battie publishes *Treatise on Madness.*

**ITALY**
**1761** Morgagni's (1682-1771) *De sedibus.*

**RUSSIA**
**1762-96** Reign of Catherine II (the Great) of Russia.

**BRITAIN**
**1763** Joseph Black (1728-1799) differentiates between specific and latent heat. **1764** Spinning Jenny introduced by Hargreaves.

**EUROPE**
**1756-63** Seven Years' War. **1758** Return of Halley's comet.

**INDIA**
**1756** Black Hole of Calcutta.

**PORTUGAL**
**1755** Earthquake of Lisbon.

**USA**
**1760** Act to regulate practice of medicine in New York City.

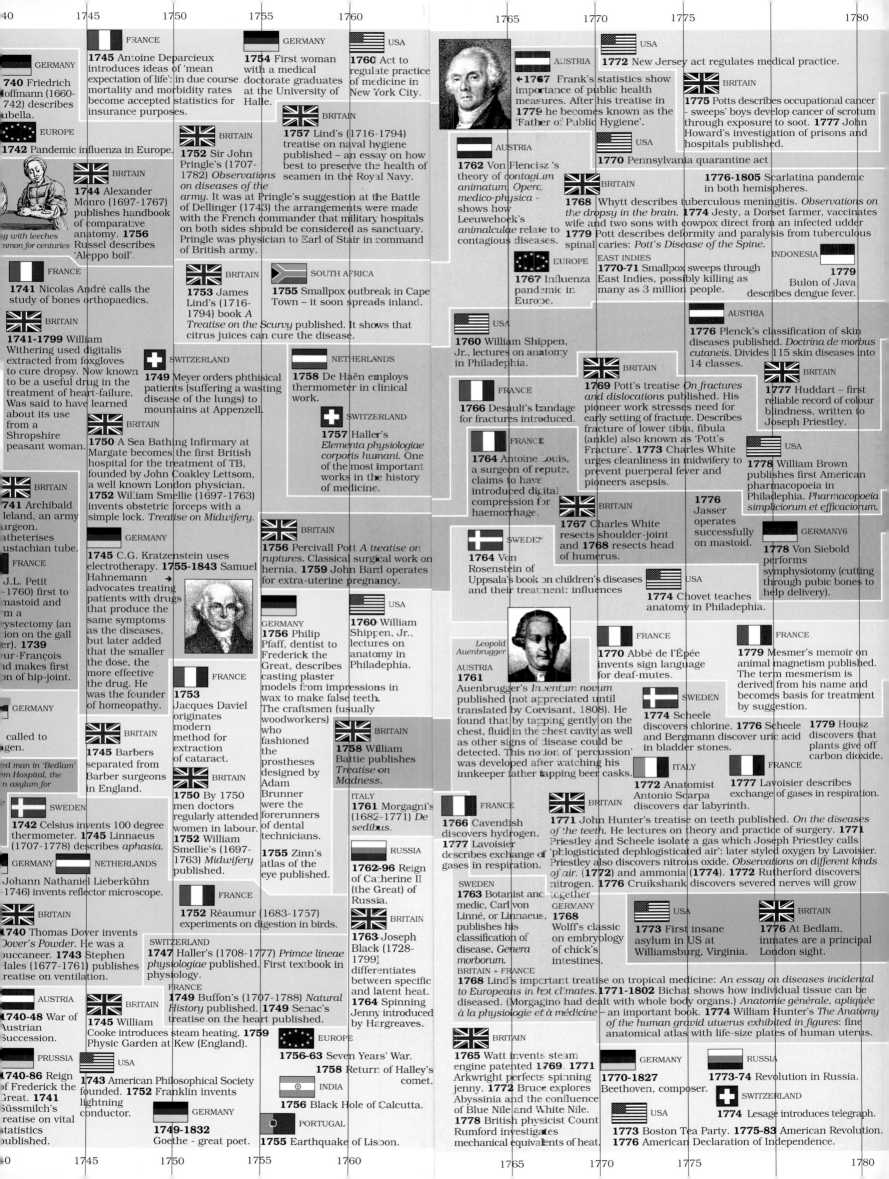

**AUSTRIA**
←**1767** Frank's statistics show importance of public health measures. After his treatise in **1779** he becomes known as the 'Father of Public Hygiene'.

**AUSTRIA**
**1762** Von Flencisz 's theory of *contagium animatum. Opera medico-physica* - shows how Leeuwehoek's *animalculae* relate to contagious diseases.

**EUROPE**
**1767** Influenza pandemic in Europe.

**USA**
**1760** William Shippen, Jr., lectures on anatomy in Philadelphia.

**FRANCE**
**1766** Desault's bandage for fractures introduced.

**FRANCE**
**1764** Antoine Louis, a surgeon of repute, claims to have introduced digital compression for haemorrhage.

**SWEDEN**
**1764** Von Rosenstein of Uppsala's book on children's diseases and their treatment: influences

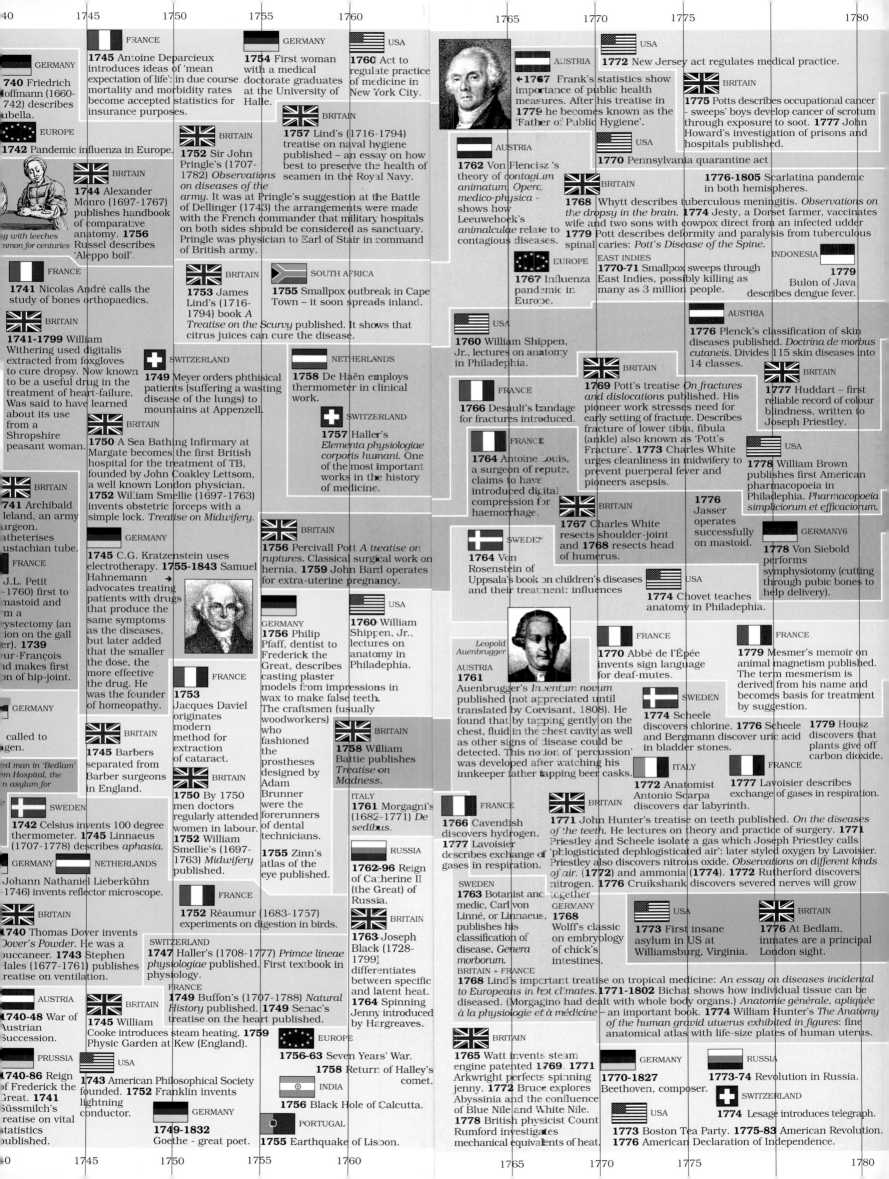

*Leopold Auenbrugger*
**AUSTRIA**
**1761** Auenbrugger's *Inventum novum* published (not appreciated until translated by Corvisant, 1808). He found that by tapping gently on the chest, fluid in the chest cavity as well as other signs of disease could be detected. This notion of 'percussion' was developed after watching his innkeeper father tapping beer casks.

**FRANCE**
**1766** Cavendish discovers hydrogen. **1777** Lavoisier describes exchange of gases in respiration.

**SWEDEN**
**1763** Botanist and medic, Carl von Linné, or Linnaeus, publishes his classification of disease, *Genera morborum.*

**GERMANY**
**1768** Wolff's classic on embryology of chick's intestines.

**BRITAIN + FRANCE**
**1768** Lind's important treatise on tropical medicine: *An essay on diseases incidental to Europeans in hot climates*. **1771-1802** Bichat shows how individual tissue can be diseased. (Morgagno had dealt with whole body organs.) *Anatomie générale, apliquée à la physiologie et à médicine* – an important book. **1774** William Hunter's *The Anatomy of the human gravid uterus exhibited in figures*: fine anatomical atlas with life-size plates of human uterus.

**BRITAIN**
**1765** Watt invents steam engine patented **1769**. **1771** Arkwright perfects spinning jenny. **1772** Bruce explores Abyssinia and the confluence of Blue Nile and White Nile. **1778** British physicist Count Rumford investigates mechanical equivalent of heat.

**USA**
**1772** New Jersey act regulates medical practice.

**BRITAIN**
**1775** Potts describes occupational cancer - sweeps' boys develop cancer of scrotum through exposure to soot. **1777** John Howard's investigation of prisons and hospitals published.

**USA**
**1770** Pennsylvania quarantine act

**1776-1805** Scarlatina pandemic in both hemispheres.

**BRITAIN**
**1768** Whytt describes tuberculous meningitis. *Observations on the dropsy in the brain.* **1774** Jesty, a Dorset farmer, vaccinates wife and two sons with cowpox direct from an infected udder **1779** Pott describes deformity and paralysis from tuberculous spinal caries: *Pott's Disease of the Spine.*

**EAST INDIES**
**1770-71** Smallpox sweeps through East Indies, possibly killing as many as 3 million people.

**INDONESIA**
**1779** Bulon of Java describes dengue fever.

**AUSTRIA**
**1776** Plenck's classification of skin diseases published. *Doctrina de morbus cutaneis.* Divides 115 skin diseases into 14 classes.

**BRITAIN**
**1769** Pott's treatise *On fractures and dislocations* published. His pioneer work stresses need for early setting of fracture. Describes fracture of lower tibia, fibula (ankle) also known as 'Pott's Fracture'. **1773** Charles White urges cleanliness in midwifery to prevent puerperal fever and pioneers asepsis.

**BRITAIN**
**1777** Huddart – first reliable record of colour blindness, written to Joseph Priestley.

**USA**
**1778** William Brown publishes first American pharmacopoeia in Philadelphia. *Pharmacopoeia simpliciorum et efficaciorum.*

**BRITAIN**
**1767** Charles White resects shoulder-joint and **1768** resects head of humerus.

**1776** Jasser operates successfully on mastoid.

**GERMANY6**
**1778** Von Siebold performs symphysiotomy (cutting through pubic bones to help delivery).

**USA**
**1774** Chovet teaches anatomy in Philadelphia.

**FRANCE**
**1770** Abbé de l'Épée invents sign language for deaf-mutes.

**FRANCE**
**1779** Mesmer's memoir on animal magnetism published. The term mesmerism is derived from his name and becomes basis for treatment by suggestion.

**SWEDEN**
**1774** Scheele discovers chlorine. **1776** Scheele and Bergmann discover uric acid in bladder stones.

**1779** Housz discovers that plants give off carbon dioxide.

**ITALY**
**1772** Anatomist Antonio Scarpa discovers ear labyrinth.

**FRANCE**
**1777** Lavoisier describes exchange of gases in respiration.

**BRITAIN**
**1771** John Hunter's treatise on teeth published. *On the diseases of the teeth.* He lectures on theory and practice of surgery. **1771** Priestley and Scheele isolate a gas which Joseph Priestley calls 'phlogisticated dephlogisticated air': later styled oxygen by Lavoisier. Priestley also discovers nitrous oxide. *Observations on different kinds of air.* (**1772**) and ammonia (**1774**). **1772** Rutherford discovers nitrogen. **1776** Cruikshank discovers severed nerves will grow together

**USA**
**1773** First insane asylum in US at Williamsburg, Virginia.

**BRITAIN**
**1776** At Bedlam, inmates are a principal London sight.

**GERMANY**
**1770-1827** Beethoven, composer.

**RUSSIA**
**1773-74** Revolution in Russia.

**SWITZERLAND**
**1774** Lesage introduces telegraph.

**USA**
**1773** Boston Tea Party. **1775-83** American Revolution. **1776** American Declaration of Independence.

## Society

**BRITAIN 1800s** Industrial Revolution: many work in difficult conditions in factories and

**BRITAIN 1785** Physician to British Fleet, Sir Gilbert Blane publishes *Observations on diseases incident to seamen*. A supporter of Lind, he effectively improved conditions in the Navy. **1796** Jenner vaccinates James Phipps with material from a cowpox sore **1798** Jenner's *Inquiry* published. **1799** De Carro introduces Jennerian vaccination

**USA 1799** Congress passes quarantine act. **1800** Waterhouse introduces Jennerian vaccination in New England.

**BRITAIN & USA Early 19th century** Many water supp polluted. Sewage finds its way from ces into wells and waterways. Garbage pol the streets or is in open dumps.

*Drink carried many such a*

## Public health

**Disease**

**BRITAIN 1786** Lettsom describes drug habit and alcoholism.

**EUROPE 1788** Influenza pandemic.

**USA 1793** Carey describes yellow fever epidemic in Philadelphia. **1796** Yellow fever in Boston. **1797-99** Yellow fever in Philadelphia.

**BRITAIN 1803** Percival publishes code of medical ethics. UK and USA medical professions adopt much of this in their ethical works.

**GERMANY 1807** Compulsory vaccination introduced in Bavaria and He

**BRITAIN 1786** John Hunter publishes *A Treatise on the Venereal Disease*. Hunter inoculated himself with pus from a patient with gonorrhea, who also had syphilis: this Hunter did not know. When Hunter developed a syphilitic chancre (sore) he thought it confirmed his theory that both diseases were caused by the same pathogen – a confusion not cleared up until 50 years later!

**BRITAIN 1798-1808** Willan's treatise on skin diseases published. *On cutaneous diseases*.

**ITALY 1804** Scarpa describes arteriosclerosis (hardening of arteries).

## Diagnosis

**BRITAIN 1793** Bell differentiates between gonorrhea and syphilis. **1793** Baillie's *Morbid Anatomy* published, covering some of the most important parts of the human body. **1798** Dalton describes colour blindness.

**ITALY 1787** Paolo Mascagni publishes atlas of the lymphatics. **1794** Antonio Scarpa's *Tabulae nevrologicae* illustrates his important work on nerves of the heart.

**FRANCE 1800** founder of modern histology and tissue pathology, Bichat publishes *Traité des membranes*. **1810-19** Gall and Spurzheim publish extraordinary treatise on the nervous system. They teach that the and irregularities of the skull were projections of the underlying brain an indicate mental characteristics. Gives rise to popular pseudo-science of phren

**BRITAIN 1809** Allan Burns descr various cardiac conditi

## Treatment

**BRITAIN 1785** Withering publishes *An account of the foxglove* about his use of digitalis to cure dropsy **1794** John Hunter publishes *Treatise on the blood inflammation and gunshot wounds*. **1797** Currie publishes reports on hydrotherapy in typhoid fever. **1797** Rollo advocates meat diet in diabetes.

*Foxglove – source of digitalis: its effects were explored by William Withering*

**FRANCE 19th century** Bloodletting still a popular treatment. 40 million leeches imported into France in one year.

*Dominique-Jean Larrey could amputate a leg in 15 seconds*

**FRANCE 1812** Napoleon's surgeon, Baron La first uses local anaesthesia. During retreat from Moscow he amputates painlessly after freezing them.

**USA 1791-99** Baynham of Virginia operates for extra-uterine pregnancy.

**FRANCE 1793-1815** Treatment of wounded in the Napoleonic wars leads to advances in surgery. A great military surgeon, present at all Napoleon's battles, Dominique-Jean Larrey performs over 200 amputations in 24 hours during Russian campaign. He develops 'flying ambulances' - wagons to carry stretchers during battle and a transport system to bring speedier attention to wounded. **1794** Chemist, Lavoisier, guillotined in French Revolution.

**BRITAIN 1794** John Hunter describes transplantation of animal tissues.

**USA 1809** McDowell of Kentuck performs ovariotomy (remov ovary) with help of his neph Mrs Crawford arrives for he operation resting her large tu (at first believed to be a pregn on the horn of her horse's sa

## Surgery

**AUSTRIA 1783** Austria separates surgeons from barbers.

**USA 1790** Medical journal published in New York.

*Dominique-Jean Larrey*

**BRITAIN 1812** Miranda Stewart B dressed as a man, attends Edinburgh University as J Barrie and qualifies as a doctor in 1812, aged 15. After se with the Duke of Wellington and becoming assistant su at the Battle of Waterloo in 1815, she becomes Insp General in 1858. Only after her death was it discovered James Barrie was a wo

## Healers and teachers

**BRITAIN 1781** Henry Cavendish (born 1731 in France, died in Britain) determines composition of water; **1784** he discovers hydrogen. **1785** Withering's treatise on the foxglove **1785** John Hunter discovers collateral circulation and introduces proximal ligation (tying up a bleeding artery) in aneurysm (a swelling of the artery). This closing off of arteries saves many limbs from amputation. **1789** John Hunter describes intussusception, a form of bowel obstruction. **1797** Wollaston discovers uric acid in gouty joints. *On gouty and urinary conditions*.

**BRITAIN 1801** Thomas Young describes astigmatism.

**EUROPE 1800s** Silver amalgam, a refinement of filling ma in dentistry, was first discovered by Europeans.

## Related skills and sciences

## Inventions and discoveries

**USA 1780** Benjamin Franklin invents bifocal lenses.

**ITALY 1784** Cotugno discovers cerebro-spinal fluid.

**USA 1792** Cotton gin (Eli Whitney).

**BRITAIN 1800** Sir Humphry Davy discovers anaesthetic effect of nitrous oxide 'laughing gas' and suggests its use during surgical operations – not effected until 1804. **1811** Sir Charles Bell describe motor functions of spinal nerve-roots. *Idea of a new anatomy of the brain*. **18 Davy knighted. Among his discoveries are sodium, potassium, boron and acety He investigated many chemical reactions, and invented miner's safety lamp.

**GERMANY 1805** Sertürner isolates morphine.

## Mental health

**GERMANY 1781** Kant's *Critique of Pure Reason* published.

**FRANCE ←1783-85** Chemist, Lavoisier decomposes water, proves that combustion needs only oxygen, and overthrows theory of phlogiston (an imaginary fire element). **1789-99** French Revolution.

**BRITAIN 1798** Malthus' *Essay on Population* **1802** Heberden's *Commentaries*: Rolleston said it had the distinction of being last important treatise written in Latin.

**POLAND/GERMANY 1791** Soemmering publishes first volume of his anatomy.

**GERMANY 1792-1821** Frank's *De curandis hominum morbis epitome* published in 7 volumes.

**BRITAIN 1798** John Haslam describes general paralysis of the insane. *Observations on insanity* – now known to be due to syphilis.

**1794** Gumpertz publishes Greek text of Asclepiades.

**USA 1797** Medical Repository (New York) published.

**FRANCE 1801** Pinel publishes psychiatric treatise. He is credited with reforming the treatment of the insane from prison-like conditions to hospital-type care.

**FRANCE 1800** Cuvier's *Comparative Anatomy* published.

**FRANCE 1801** Bichat's *Anatomie générale* published. He revolutionised descriptive anatomy. **1824** Flourens publishes work on cerebral physiology.

**USA 1812** Rush write American book o psychiatry, *Medic inquiries and observations upo diseases of the m*

## Printing and publishing

**BRITAIN 1785** Cartwright invents power loom. **1787** Voyage of the *Bounty* under Lieutenant Bligh. **1792** Murdock introduces gas lighting to Britain. **1794** Erasmus Darwin's *Zoonomia* published. A system of pathology and a treatise on generation. Grandfather of Charles Darwin. **1795** Mungo Park explores River Niger.

*Many plants were discovered on Captain Cook's voyages*

**FRANCE 1791** Dr Guillotin invents guillotine. **1792** Establishment of French Republic **1793-94** Reign of Terror in France. **1798** Gas lighting introduced. **1799-1804** Napoleon First Consul. **1804-15** Napoleon Emperor of the French.

**BRITAIN 1797** Last invasion of mainland Britain. French troops land in Wales. **1804** Dalton states atomic theory. **1804** First railway engine. **1810** Davy analyses corrosive sublimate. **1814** Stephenson's first locomotive.

**BE 1815** Bat Waterloo.

## World events and inventions

**BRITAIN 1768-79** Captain James Cook's three voyages to the Pacific. **1769** Charts coasts of New Zealand and eastern Australia. **1770** Lands at Botany Bay, Australia. **1773** Crosses Antarctic Circle. **1774** Charts much of Pacific. **1778** Discovers Hawaiian Islands, surveys Bering Straits.

**ITALY 1792** Volta constructs Voltaic pile. **1792** Galvani's essay on animal electricity published.

*Napoleon Bonaparte*

**1796-1815** Napoleonic Wars.

**ITALY 1800** Electric battery introduced by Volta.

**USA 1789** George Washington President. **1790** George Vancouver explores the coast of north-west America. **1801** Jefferson becomes President. **1806** Fulton invents steamboat.

**1806** End of Holy Roman Empire.

**SPAIN 1808-14** The Peninsular War.

**1805** Battle of Trafalgar.

**1809** Soemmerring invents electric telegraph.

**GE 1815** Ger Confedera

**1815** Da invents lamp for miners.

Apothecaries Act

**BRITAIN**
**1832** Anatomy Act passed

**BRITAIN**
**1837** Introduction of registration of deaths introduced in England and Wales.

**FRANCE**
**1826** Laënnec gives classical description of bronchitis and other thoracic diseases. **1835** Cruveilhier (1791-1874) describes disseminated sclerosis (now known as multiple sclerosis).

**BRITAIN**
**1835** Malcolmson describes beri-beri. **1836** Richard Bright describes acute yellow atrophy of liver. Investigates mechanism of urinary secretion.

**BRITAIN**
**1848** Public Health Act creates general and local boards of health.

**1840's** England pioneers principles and practices of public health, passing the Public Health Acts, which bring about cleaner water and mains drainage. **1842** Chadwick's report demonstrates link between environmental conditions and public health.

**FRANCE**
**1826** Dupuytren describes congenital dislocation of hip-joint. Very important in anatomy, and pathology, he also performs daring feats of surgery and devises ingenious instruments.

**USA**
**1832** Cholera spreads out to circle the globe, from Asia to Europe and then the USA where there are 3 outbreaks during century. **1837** Gerhard shows that typhus and typhoid are separate diseases.

**1840** Basedow describes syndromes of exophthalmic goitre – eye protrusion, neck swelling, palpitations – known in UK as Grave's Disease.

**BELGIUM**
**1852** International Congress of Hygiene.

_John Snow_

**BRITAIN**
**1849** Addison describes pernicious anaemia and a disease of the adrenals – Addison's Anaemia and Addison's

**-30** Pandemic of a: first of many this ry, it spreads from and China through pe and USA.

**USA**
**1833** William Beaumont publishes experiments on digestion.

**1837** Schönlein's _Peliosis Rheumatica_ describes skin condition of purpura, now known by his name.

**AUSTRIA**
**1847** Semmelweis shows septicaemia to be cause of puerperal fever. In 1861 he publishes book on childhood fever.

**BRITAIN**
**1854** 1,400 cases of cholera in London; 618 deaths. John Snow ended the epidemic by demonstrating that only those who drank from the Broad Street water pump contracted the disease. This pump was closed down and the outbreak ceased.

**USA**
**1821-1825** William Beaumont treats a war patient evidently dying of a close shotgun blast. He survives with permanent exterior opening to his stomach. He made studies of gastric juices on this patient.

**BRITAIN**
**1827** Richard Bright describes disease of the kidney since known as 'Bright's Disease'.

**GERMANY**
**1845** Virchow and Bennett describe leukemia.

**NORWAY**
**1849** Danielssen and Boeck publish studies on leprosy, providing impetus for a national, government-sponsored research centre.

**GERMANY**
**1837** Schwann discovers yeast cell. Regarded by many as founder of germ theory of putrification and fermentation. **1837** Jacob Henle describes epithelial tissues of skin and intestine. Modern knowledge of this starts here: possibly contributed as much to microscopic anatomy as Vesalius did for gross anatomy.

**AUSTRIA**
**1839** Skoda's treatise on percussion and auscultation lays groundwork for diagnosis today.

**GERMANY**
**1850** Helmholtz measures the velocity of the nerve current. **1851** Ludwig investigate nerves of salivary secretion. **1858** Rudolf Virchow's (1821-1902) publishes _Die Cellular Pathologie_: foundation of cellular pathology.

**FRANCE**
**1846** Bernard describes digestive function of pancreas, in **1848** discovers glycogenic function of the liver in sugar metabolism, in **1849** produces diabetes by puncture of the fourth ventricle and in **1851** describes vasomotor function of sympathetic nervous system. In **1854** he discovers function of vaso-dilator nerves of brain.

**FRANCE**
**1820** Coindet uses odine in goiter. **1822** Magendie demonstrates Bell's law of spinal nerve roots.

**BRITAIN**
**1828** Blundell reports first human-to-human blood transfusion which patient survives.

**ITALY**
**1830** Priessnitz, a Silesian peasant, is run over by a wagon and given up as a hopeless case. Using wet compresses and drinking vast amounts of water he recovers and institutes his 'water cure for disease'.

**IRELAND**
**1835** Robert James Graves classical account of exophthalmic goitre now known as Graves Disease. **1845** Francis Rynd invents an instrument to give hypodermic infusions.

**FRANCE**
**1838** Epileptic children in Paris were removed from Hospital of the Incurably Ill to another location and given some education.

**IRELAND**
**1845** Francis Rynd invents an instrument to give hypodermic infusions.

**RUSSIA**
**1852** Pirogoff employs frozen sections in his _Anatome topigraphica_.

**BRITAIN**
**1827** Lord Lister born. **1832** British Medical Association founded.

_Joseph Lister_

**NETHERLANDS**
Reimar introduces n sections.

**USA**
**1842** Long operates with ether anesthesia. **1846** William Thomas Morton uses ether to put patient to sleep during dental operation. Demonstrates this at Massachusetts General Hospital. **1850** William Detmold opens abscess of the brain.

_Morton using ether on a patient_
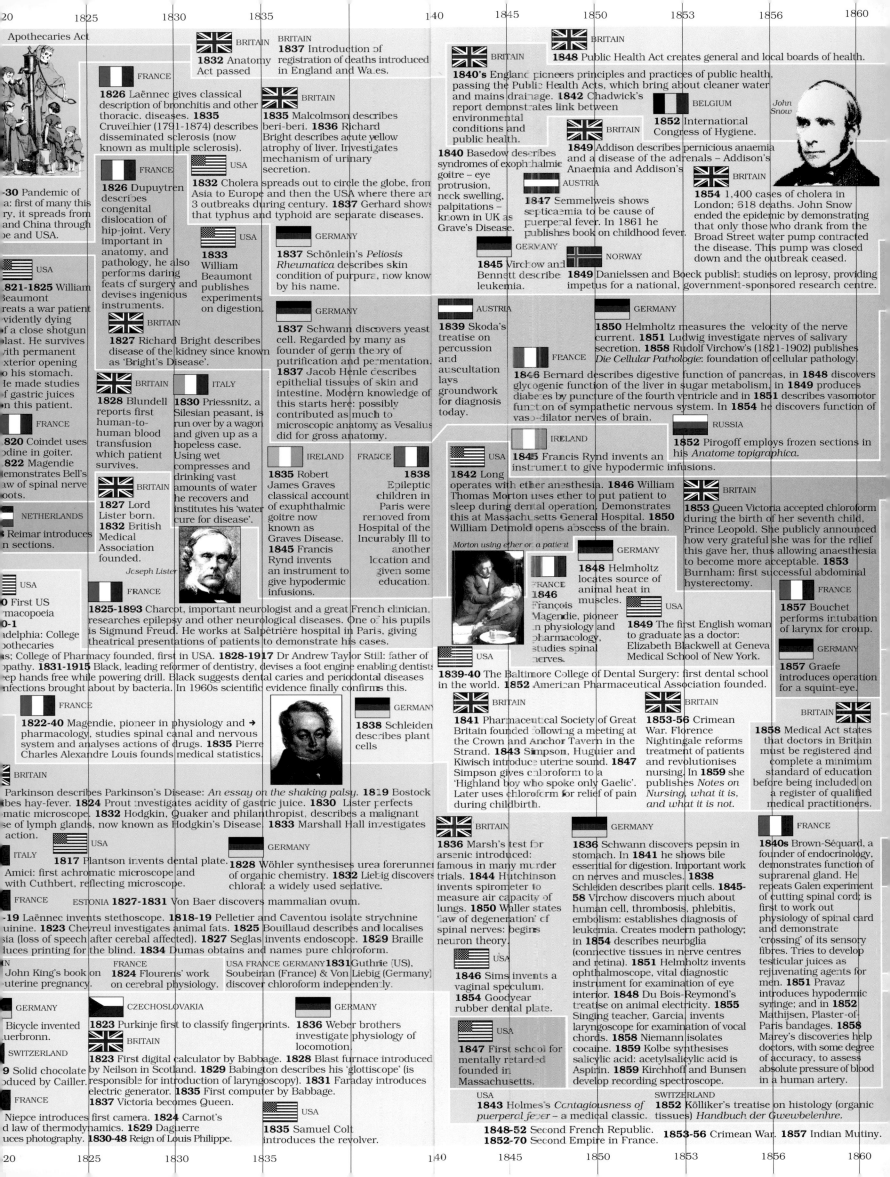

**GERMANY**
**1848** Helmholtz locates source of animal heat in muscles.

**BRITAIN**
**1853** Queen Victoria accepted chloroform during the birth of her seventh child, Prince Leopold. She publicly announced how very grateful she was for the relief this gave her, thus allowing anaesthesia to become more acceptable. **1853** Burnham: first successful abdominal hysterectomy.

**USA**
First US macopoeia 0-1 delphia: College pothecaries; College of Pharmacy founded, first in USA. **1828-1917** Dr Andrew Taylor Still: father of opathy. **1831-1915** Black, leading reformer of dentistry, devises a foot engine enabling dentists ep hands free while powering drill. Black suggests dental caries and periodontal diseases nfections brought about by bacteria. In 1960s scientific evidence finally confirms this.

**1825-1893** Charcot, important neurologist and a great French clinician, researches epilepsy and other neurological diseases. One of his pupils is Sigmund Freud. He works at Salpêtrière hospital in Paris, giving theatrical presentations of patients to demonstrate his cases.

**FRANCE**
**1846** François Magendie, pioneer in physiology and pharmacology, studies spinal nerves.

**USA**
**1849** The first English woman to graduate as a doctor: Elizabeth Blackwell at Geneva Medical School of New York.

**FRANCE**
**1857** Bouchet performs intubation of larynx for croup.

**FRANCE**
**1822-40** Magendie, pioneer in physiology and → pharmacology, studies spinal canal and nervous system and analyses actions of drugs. **1835** Pierre Charles Alexandre Louis founds medical statistics.

**GERMANY**
**1838** Schleiden describes plant cells

**USA**
**1839-40** The Baltimore College of Dental Surgery: first dental school in the world. **1852** American Pharmaceutical Association founded.

**GERMANY**
**1857** Graefe introduces operation for a squint-eye.

**BRITAIN**
Parkinson describes Parkinson's Disease: _An essay on the shaking palsy._ **1819** Bostock ibes hay-fever. **1824** Prout investigates acidity of gastric juice. **1830** Lister perfects matic microscope. **1832** Hodgkin, Quaker and philanthropist, describes a malignant se of lymph glands, now known as Hodgkin's Disease. **1833** Marshall Hall investigates action.

**BRITAIN**
**1841** Pharmaceutical Society of Great Britain founded following a meeting at the Crown and Anchor Tavern in the Strand. **1843** Simpson, Huguier and Kiwisch introduce uterine sound. **1847** Simpson gives chloroform to a 'Highland boy who spoke only Gaelic'. Later uses chloroform for relief of pain during childbirth.

**BRITAIN**
**1853-56** Crimean War. Florence Nightingale reforms treatment of patients and revolutionises nursing. In **1859** she publishes _Notes on Nursing, what it is, and what it is not._

**BRITAIN**
**1858** Medical Act states that doctors in Britain must be registered and complete a minimum standard of education before being included on a register of qualified medical practitioners.

**ITALY**
Amici: first achromatic microscope and with Cuthbert, reflecting microscope.

**USA**
**1817** Plantson invents dental plate.

**GERMANY**
**1828** Wöhler synthesises urea forerunner of organic chemistry. **1832** Liebig discovers chloral: a widely used sedative.

**BRITAIN**
**1836** Marsh's test for arsenic introduced: famous in many murder trials. **1844** Hutchinson invents spirometer to measure air capacity of lungs. **1850** Waller states 'law of degeneration' of spinal nerves: begins neuron theory.

**GERMANY**
**1836** Schwann discovers pepsin in stomach. **1841** he shows bile essential for digestion. Important work on nerves and muscles. **1838** Schleiden describes plant cells. **1845-58** Virchow discovers much about human cell, thrombosis, phlebitis, embolism: establishes diagnosis of leukemia. Creates modern pathology; in **1854** describes neuroglia (connective tissues in nerve centres and retina). **1851** Helmholtz invents ophthalmoscope, vital diagnostic instrument for examination of eye interior. **1848** Du Bois-Reymond's treatise on animal electricity. **1855** Singing teacher, Garcia, invents laryngoscope for examination of vocal chords. **1858** Niemann isolates cocaine. **1859** Kolbe synthesises salicylic acid: acetylsalicylic acid is Aspirin. **1859** Kirchhoff and Bunsen develop recording spectroscope.

**FRANCE**
**1840s** Brown-Séquard, a founder of endocrinology, demonstrates function of suprarenal gland. He repeats Galen experiment of cutting spinal cord; is first to work out physiology of spinal cord and demonstrate 'crossing' of its sensory fibres. Tries to develop testicular juices as rejuvenating agents for men. **1851** Pravaz introduces hypodermic syringe; and in **1852** Mathijsen, Plaster-of-Paris bandages. **1858** Marey's discoveries help doctors, with some degree of accuracy, to assess absolute pressure of blood in a human artery.

**FRANCE**
**1824** Flourens' work on cerebral physiology.

**USA FRANCE GERMANY 1831** Guthrie (US), Soubeiran (France) & Von Liebig (Germany) discover chloroform independently.

**USA**
**1846** Sims invents a vaginal speculum. **1854** Goodyear rubber dental plate.

ESTONIA **1827-1831** Von Baer discovers mammalian ovum.

**-19** Laënnec invents stethoscope. **1818-19** Pelletier and Caventou isolate strychnine uinine. **1823** Chevreul investigates animal fats. **1825** Bouillaud describes and localises sia (loss of speech after cerebal affected). **1827** Seglas invents endoscope. **1829** Braille luces printing for the blind. **1834** Dumas obtains and names pure chloroform.

**CZECHOSLOVAKIA**
**1823** Purkinje first to classify fingerprints.

**GERMANY**
**1836** Weber brothers investigate physiology of locomotion.

**USA**
**1847** First school for mentally retarded founded in Massachusetts.

John King's book on uterine pregnancy.

Bicycle invented uerbronn.

SWITZERLAND
9 Solid chocolate duced by Cailler.

**BRITAIN**
**1823** First digital calculator by Babbage. **1828** Blast furnace introduced by Neilson in Scotland. **1829** Babington describes his 'glottiscope' (is responsible for introduction of laryngoscopy). **1831** Faraday introduces electric generator. **1835** First computer by Babbage. **1837** Victoria becomes Queen.

**FRANCE**
Niepce introduces first camera. **1824** Carnot's d law of thermodynamics. **1829** Daguerre uces photography. **1830-48** Reign of Louis Philippe.

**USA**
**1835** Samuel Colt introduces the revolver.

**USA**
**1843** Holmes's _Contagiousness of puerperal fever_ – a medical classic.

**SWITZERLAND**
**1852** Kölliker's treatise on histology (organic tissues) _Handbuch der Gwewbelenhre._

**1848-52** Second French Republic.
**1852-70** Second Empire in France.

**1853-56** Crimean War. **1857** Indian Mutiny.

**Society**

1868 UK Pharmacy Art

GERMANY

FRANCE 1874 *Loi Roussel* enacted for the protection of infants.

USA — EUROPE

1890s Pharmaceutical industry advertisemen appear. Beechams's Pills spread from Britain to

**Public health**

CHOLERA. DUDLEY BOARD OF HEALTH

1866 Voit (1831-1908) establishes first hygienic laboratory in Munich. 1869 Virchow (1821-1902) urges medical inspection of schools. 1873 Revaccination compulsory. 1875 Meat inspection compulsory.

BRITAIN 1872 Infant life protection act passed in England. 1875 Public Health Act – will remain charter of English public health for next 60 years. 1889 Infectious Diseases (Notification) Act in England and Wales. 1896 Dibdin introduces biological purification of sewage.

BAYER PHARMACEUTICAL PRODUCTS. Send for samples and Literature to FARBENFABRIKEN OF ELBERFELD CO. 40 STONE STREET, NEW YORK.

GERMANY 1891 Institute for Infectious Diseases in Berlin opens.

BRITAIN 1897-98 Ross discover parasite responsible fo malaria; and role of mosquito in bird malar

**Disease**

FRANCE

1860 Menière describes aural vertigo, a form of severe giddiness known as Menière's Disease. 1863 Pasteur investigates silkworm disease which was affecting economy of France. 1865 Villemin demonstrates that TB is due to a specific agent, which he called a germ.

SWEDEN 1881 Medin discovers epidemic nature of poliomyelitis.

FRANCE 1880 Laveran first sees parasite of malaria fever.

Robert Koch

USA 1892 Welch and Nuttall discover gas gangrene bacillus. 1899 Lazear and others establish transmissi yellow fever by mosquito. *Aëdes aegypti etiology of yellow fever.* Lazear dies from y fever after accidental mosquito bite.

JAPAN 1897 Shiga discovers dysentery bacillus.

GERMANY Discoveries: 1883 Klebs – diphtheria bacillus. 1883 Koch – cholera bac 1884 Nicolaier – tetanus bacillus. 1882 Koch – tubercle ba

**Diagnosis**

USA 1861-65 American Civil War. Many outbreaks of communicable diseases.

FRANCE 1861 Broca reports that speech control is located in left frontal lobe of brain. 1873 Cuignet introduces retinoscopy.

BRITAIN 1875 Sir Thomas Barlow describes infantile scurvy, Barlow's Disease.

1880 Balfour's *Treatise on comparative embryology.* Classical summary of previous knowledge. 1880 Sir William Richard Gowers, one of founders of modern neurology: *Diagnosis of Diseases of the Spi.nal Chord.*

USA 1897 Medical student, Cannon uses solution radio-opaque bismuth a diagnostic meal to outline stomach.

**Treatment**

GERMANY 1860 Von Tröltsch devises first modern mastoid operation. 1862 V Bruns performs first operation with laryngoscope. Lewin also did this in the same year. 1869 Esmarch introduces india rubber bandage devised to provide bloodless field for limb surgery. 1870 Gustav Simon reports successful planned removal of kidney. 1873 Schwartze and Eysell revise mastoid operation.

GERMANY 1868 Wunderlich's *Das Verhalten Eigen wasme in Krankeiten:* classical work on temperature in disease – founded use of clinical thermometer.

USA 1875 Mitchell introduces rest cure for treatment of nervous diseases.

GERMANY 1877 Cohnheim makes successful inoculation of tuberculosis in rabbit's eye. 1890 Behring treats diphtheria with antitoxin. 1893 A chemist markets aspirin, using it to treat rheumatism. 1898 Dreser introduces aspirin into medicine.

GERMANY/AUSTRIA 1873 Billroth excises the larynx.

CZECHOSLOVAKIA 1867 Rokitansky performs nearly 60,000 autopsies in 50 years.

BRITAIN 1874 Tait carries out first hysterectomy; in 1879 first *successful* cholecsytectomy (cutting out of a gall bladder) and in 1883 operates successfully for extra-uterine (ectopic) pregnancy. 1885 Bennett and Sir Rickman Godlee credited with first successful removal of a brain tumour. 1887 Gowers and Horsley operate on spinal cord. Sir Victor Horsley was a pioneer brain surgeon who removed spinal cord tumours. 1894 Sir William Arbuthnot Lane introduces pinning of fractures but metals used were often rejected by the body.

GER 1891 Quincke popularises lumbar puncture.

FRANCE 1883 Pasteur vaccinates against anthrax and in 1885-6 deve first effective vaccine against rabies: *Méthode pour prévenir la*

**Surgery**

FRANCE 1862 Artery clamps invented.

BRITAIN 1865 First real test of Lister's antiseptic procedures performed in treatment of compound fracture. 1872 Artery clamps developed by Wells.

AUSTRIA 1879 Czerny describes vaginal route for total hystorectomy.

USA 1884 Koller uses cocaine in eye surgery. 1885 Halsted first experiments on local infiltration anaesthesia and in 1890 introduces rubber gloves for surgery at Johns Hopkins.

**Healers and teachers**

BRITAIN 1865 Elizabeth Garrett Anderson obtains Diploma of Society of Apothecaries, London.

**Related skills and sciences**

NETHERLANDS 1860 Donders who studied many eye defects, introduces spectacles for astigmatism and in 1862 publishes studies on astigmatism and presbyopia.

ITALY 1876 Lombroso's doctrine of 'criminal type'. *L'uomo delinquente.*

GERMANY 1878 Von Volkmann successfully removes a cancer of the rectum and Freund excises a cance uterus. 1881 Billroth resects (cuts away) the pylorus (opening of stomach into duodenum cancer. 1882 Sänger describes 'classic Caesarean section'. 1886 Von Bergmann introduc steam sterilisation in surgery. 1894 Schleich develops infiltration anesthesia. 1895 Kirst devises direct vision laryngoscopy. 1898 Killian uses direct bronchoscopy.

BRITAIN 1863 Harrington invents clockwork dental drill.

AUSTRIA 1865 Gregor Mendel publishes experiments on plant hybrids which form basis of science of genetics. These were overlooked and neglected until 1900.

Gregor Mendel

BRITAIN 1886 An amendment to the Medical Act makes midwifery training (however derisory) part of doctors' training.

USA — CANADA 1895 Chiropractic manipula of joints introduced by Palm

**Inventions and discoveries**

FRANCE 1861 Pasteur discovers anaerobic bacteria and in 1863 that bacteria are destroyed by heat; he invents pasteurisation. 1867 Claude Bernard founder of experimental physiology, establishes principle of homeostasis, that red blood corpuscles carry oxygen, discovers much about the functions of internal organs and digestion, and links pancreas to diabetes.

AUSTRIA 1865 Mendel's theory of inheritance shows that genes carry sets of instructions from parents to offspring.

JAPAN GERMANY 1890 Von Behring and Kitasato discover diphtheria and tetanus antitoxins and provide basis for serotherapy.

RUSSIA 1892 Ivanovski's work on tobacco mosaic disease develops knowledge of viruses.

USA 1897-98 Walter B. Car discovers barium suspen show up alimentary can x-ray plate.

AUSTRIA Gärtner uses tonometer in for measuring blood pressu means of finger

GERMANY 1861 Schultze defines protoplasm and cell. 1862 Felix Hoppe Seyler discovers haemoglobin. 1863 Preparation of barbituric acid (barbiturates) by Baeyer. 1867 Kussmaul introduces intubation of stomach. 1870 Fritsch and Hitzig investigate localisation of functions of brain. 1871 Weigert stains bacteria with carmine. 1874 Ehrlich introduces dried blood smears and improves stain methods.

RUSSIA 1867 Ivan Petrovich Pavlov famous for his dogs! He contributed to understanding of conditioned reflexes. His work was misused for brain washing techniques.

BRITAIN 1873-4 Sir William Gull describes myxedoema (thyroid deficiency) and anorexia nervosa. 1877 Sir Patrick Manson shows mosquitoes transmit *Wucheria bancrofti* as cause of filarial elephantiasis in man. First proof that infective diseases transmitted by insect vector. 1888 Nuttall discovers bactericidal powers of blood-serum. 1898 Pioneer pathologist Theobald Smith differentiates between bovine and human tubercle bacilli.

GERMAN Discoveries: 1879 Neisser – gonococcus (which causes gonorrhea). 1880 Eberth – typhoid bacillus. 1882 Koch– tubercle bacillus 1887 Weichselbaum – meningococcus 1889 Von Behring – anti-toxins. Introductions: 1876 Koch – growing anthrax bacilli on artificial media and in 1881 – plate cultures 1882 Flemming investigates cell division. 1886 Von Soxhlet – sterilised milk for infants. 1890 Koch tuberculin. 1895 Wilhelm Röntgen takes first x-ray → of his wife's hand.

JAPAN FRANCE 1894 Kitasato and Yersin discover plague bacillus.

GE FRANCE 1898-99 Dreser introduces drugs hero and aspirin into medic

**Mental health**

FRANCE 1880 Pasteur isolates streptococcus, staphylococcus and pneumococcus. 1888 Roux and Yersin investigate toxins of diphtheria. 1896 Becquerel discovers radioactivity in uranium. 1898 Pierre and Marie→ Curie discover radium.

**Printing and publishing**

BRITAIN 1864 Edmund Alexando Parkes' important *Manual of Practical Hygiene* published.

GERMANY 1867 Helmholtz (1821-1894) publishes treatise on physiological optics.

AUSTRIA 1895 Freud (with Breu publishes *Studien über Hysterie* on the revelat of the 'unconscious mi ←1900 Freud publishe *The interpretation of dreams,* which had a w influence beyond medi

**World events and inventions**

ITALY 1860 Garibaldi takes southern Italy: most of Italy united.

AUSTRIA GERMANY 1866 Seven Weeks' (Austro-Prussian) War.

EGYPT 1867 Opening of Suez Canal.

FRANCE GERMANY 1870-71 Franco-Prussian War (test of vaccination). Establishment of German Empire and French Republic.

USA 1876 Sioux Rising. 1876 Bell invents telephone. 1879 Edison's electric light bulb. 1889 Photographic film introduced by Eastman. 1898 Spanish-American War.

CHINA 1894-1945 Chinese-Japanese

FRANCE 1895 Lumière Brothers invent proje

BRITAIN 1855 David Livingstone discovers Victoria Falls. 1855 Refrigerator introduced 1859 Darwin's *Origin of Species* and in 1871 his *The Descent of Man.* USA 1846 Elias Howe (1819-1867) patents sewing machine. 1849 Walter Hunt invents the safety pin. 1849 Gold Rush in California.

SWITZERLAND 1864 Geneva Convention signed, embodying principles of the international Red Cross.

FRANCE 1858 Refrigerator introduced by Carré. 1859 First internal combustion engine.

USA/BRITAIN 1875 Stanley explores River Congo.

AFRICA 1877-78 Zulu War: famous stand at Rorke's Drift. 1884-1888 Sudan War. Gordon killed at Khartoum 1885).

GERMANY 1884 First car. 1885 Daimler's motorcycle. 1886 Benz's petrol car. 1888-1918 Kaiser Wilhem's reign.

NORWAY 1888-93 Nansen explores Greenland and tries to find North Pole.

1874 International postal service.

RUSSIA TURKEY 1877-78 Russo-Turkish War.

ITALY 1895 Marconi introduces wire telegra

SWEDEN 1895 Death of Alfred Nobel. N Prize Fund announced in his First awarded 1901.

USA
International Sanitary Bureau ...lished (later Pan-American Health ...nisation). **1906** Food and Drugs ...**1917-18** American Commission ...tigates trench fever.

USA
**1910** Law against White Slave traffic.
**1912** Public Health Services set up.
**1912** Children's Bureau established (Washington, D.C.). **1913** Supreme Court denies 'rights' of individuals when inimical to public welfare.

BRITAIN
**1919** British Ministry of Health established.

**1942** World Health Organisation (WHO) set up as an agency of the United Nations.

BRITAIN
**1948** National Health Service starts. **1948** The Kinsey report.

USA
**1938** New York is first state to pass a law requiring medical tests for US marriage licences. **1945** World's first fluoridated water supply is available in Michigan.

**1950s** DDT sprays used to kill insects.

BRITAIN
Manson's ...riments prove ...quito vector of ...ria: volunteer ...son!

USA
**1906** 'Typhoid Mary", most famous typhoid carrier, discovered. **1907** Immigrants given health check to ensure not carrying any contagious disease; unhealthy ones may be sent back home. **1910** Ricketts demonstrates woodtick as vector of Rocky Mountain Spotted Fever, which he differentiated from typhus. **1910** Flexner produces poliomyelitis experimentally. **1911** Rous transmits malignant tumour, as a filterable virus.

JAPAN
**1916** Futaki and others discover spirillum in rabite fever.

**1918-19** Influenza pandemic kills 15 million people.

**1932** Scientists announce development of first vaccine against yellow fever. **1945** A vaccine against virus A and B influenza is used on the US army for the first time.

USA
**1953** Virologist, Dr Salk, successfully tests a vaccine against polio.

BRITAIN
Dutton and Forde identify parasite of Gambian Fever: helps ...rstanding of sleeping sickness which in **1903** Bruce and Nabarro ...y is transmitted by tsetse fly. **1908** Sleeping Sickness Bureau founded. ...Bass and Johns cultivate malarial plasmodium in a test tube.

GERMANY
**1913** Schweitzer starts his grat work in Africa, building hospitals and fighting leprosy

NETHERLANDS
**1930** Chemist, Debye, uses x-rays to investigate structure of molecules.

USA
**1934** Mixter and Barr demonstrate role of intervertebral disc herniation in sciatica.

Birth control clinic 1920s

GERMANY
/05 Koch ...s bubonic ...se may have ...due to rats; ...tigates ...an fever.

NEW ZEALAND
**1906** Bancroft demonstrates dengue transmitted by mosquito bites: *Aëdes aegypti.*

TUNISIA
**1909** Nicolle shows body lice spread typhus.

GERMANY
**1912** Sudhoff opposes theory of American origin of syphilis: believes it existed in Europe pre-Columbus.

BRITAIN
**1936** Bach's flower remedies made commercially.

**1920s** Marie Stopes opens first birth-control clinic, offering free consultations and contraceptives. Examinations carried out by a midwife, and if necessary, patients are referred to the clinic's female doctor **1925** First successful insulin treatment is performed in Europe at Guys Hospital, London. **1928** Sir Alexander Fleming discovers penicillin the first antibiotic. **1940** The experiments of Florey and Chain effect a method for production of stable, solid penicillin for therapeutic use.

FRANCE
**1905** ...ychologist Alfred ...et develops a way ...sting the brain on ...ability to reason.

GERMANY
**1907** Wassermann introduces sero diagnostic test for syphilis.

BRITAIN
**1910** Marine and others suggest that goiter (enlargement of thyroid) may be prevented by taking iodine. **1915** British introduce tetanus antitoxin for all wounded soldiers.

BELGIUM
**1917** Willems early mobilisation of joint wounds changes orthopaedic practice.

CANADA
**1921** Insulin treatment for diabetes developed by Banting and Best.

*Human kidney transplants begin in the 1950s*

USA
**1928** The iron lung, developed in 1927 by US physicist Philip Drinker, is used for the first time in the USA. **1944** Waksman discovers streptomycin, a useful antibiotic effective against brucellosis and tuberculosis. **1945** Benadryl is developed to treat common allergies such as hayfever and asthma. **1950** First human kidney transplant, performed by Lawler.

DENMARK
Finsen, founder ...otorapy, ...nstrates ...peutic value of ...ctinec ray and ultra violet light.

AUSTRIA
**1907** Von Pirquet introduces TB skin test.

*Lavender*

CZECHOSLOVAKIA
**1910** Jansky demonstrates four basic blood groups A, B, AB and O.

FRANCE
**1910** Gattefossé applies lavender oil to a burn which heals quickly with little scarring: he studies therapeutic actions of plant oils. **1913** De Sandfort devises ambrine (paraffin-resin solution) treatment for burns. **1914-1918** Carrel and Dakin devise treatment of infected wounds.

ITALY
**1916** Vanghetti introduces cineplasty – using muscle above stump to activate artificial limbs.

FRANCE
**1921** Development of a vaccine against tuberculosis using non-virulent bovine bacilli by Calmette and Guérin. **1922** McCollum (and others) identify 'Vitamin D'. It promotes proper bone growth and helps combat rickets. **1924** Albert Calmette introduces BCG preventive vaccination of children against tuberculosis.

GERMANY
**1902** Formula patented for barbituric acid – used to make sleeping pills.

**1921** Nylen uses a monocular microscope during an operation on the ear for deafness.

GERMANY
**1932** Evipan, a barbiturate anaesthetic, introduced by Weese and Scharpff. **1944** Surgeon Alfred Blalock performs first successful heart operation on a newborn baby.

USA
**1952** An artificial heart is first used in an operation at Pennsylvania Hospital.

BRITAIN
**1903** Smith perfects new operation for eye cataracts.

CANADA
**1906** Surgeons perform kidney operations on animals to prove human transplants possible.

USA
**1910** X-ray machine guides a surgeon to remove a nail from the lung of a boy.

FRANCE
**1912** Professor Dastre pioneers cornea graft to restore lost eyesight.

BELGIUM
**1920** First Congress of Medical History (Antwerp).

←**1947** Gerty T. Cori is first woman to win the Nobel Prize in medicine, along with her husband Carl F. Cori, for their discovery of the process in the catalytic metabolism of glycogen.

GERMANY
**1900** Wertheim ...ntroduces radical operation for uterine ...cancer. **1904** Sauerbruch designs negative pressure chamber for chest surgery.

BRITAIN
**1914-18** Modern plastic surgery develops with Gillies pioneering use of pedicle flaps of skin from one part of body to another.

HUNGARY
**1928** Biochemist Szent-Györgyi manages to isolate vitamin C.

USA
**1950** Howard Green grows human skin for grafting from a one square millimetre amount taken from a newborn baby. This grows to an area of 60 square centimetres in 20 days.

BRITAIN
**1913** International Medical Congress

FRANCE
**1926** Pasteur Institute announces discovery of an anti-tetanus serum.

GERMANY
**1932** First electron-microscope constructed by Ruska and Knoll.

BRITAIN
**1901** In Scotland hospital beds set ...aside for first ever ante-natal care.

SWEDEN
**1911** Gullstrand receives Nobel prize for optical research.

AUSTRALIA
**1912** First ante-natal clinic opens in Sydney

AUSTRALIA
**1928** Flying doctor service is set up in Queensland.

USA
**1933** Anti-beriberi vitamin identified by Robert Williams and colleagues. **1936** Anti-beriberi vitamin produced synthetically.

USA
**1944** First eye bank is opened by Manhattan and New York hospitals. **1946** Dr Benjamin Spock publishes *Baby and Child Care* which tells parents to hug their children and follow their instincts, rather than imposing set routines and rigorous discipline.

USA
**1903** Dentists propose porcelain for fillings or crowns. **1911** First ante-natal clinic opens in Boston. **1915** Fitzgerald describes zone therapy.

FRANCE
USSR
**1937** Artificial heart by Vladimir P. Demikhov.

USA
**1950** Küss in Paris and Murray in Boston, with their colleagues, transplant first kidneys from deceased to living patients.

BELGIUM
**1905** ...rdet and Gengou ...scover bacillus of ...whooping-cough.

FRANCE
**1907** Calmette devises conjunctival test for TB. **1907** Doctors announce discovery of a serum which cures dysentery. **1912** Odin claims he has isolated and cultivated a cancer microbe.

USA
**1912** Cushing describes *The pituitary body and its disorders.*

BRITAIN
**1915** Dakin introduces new antiseptics.

BRITAIN
**1928** Hindle introduces first vaccine for immunisation against Yellow Fever. **1928** Elastoplast sticking plaster dressings first manufactured. **1938** Dodds, and others, introduce first synthetic oestrogen (stilboestrol).

AUSTRIA
**1940** Landsteiner and Wiener find an additional agglutination factor in blood, the Rh antigen, following experiments using a Rhesus monkey.

AUSTRIA
Three major blood cell groups ...and O described by Landsteiner: ...ork leads to safer transfusion.

POLAND
**1912** Funk proposes name 'Vitamine' (Vitamin) for substances that prevent deficiency diseases.

NETHERLANDS
**1942-43** First kidney dialysis machine is developed in secret for the Dutch resistance by Willem Kolff.

*DNA double helix structure*

USA
**1904** Atwater invents respiration calorimeter.

Ehrlich tests Salvarson in treatment of syphilis: regarded as birth of chemotherapy.

JAPAN
**1913** Noguchi demonstrates *Spirochaete pallida* in brains of syphilitic patients. Dies of Yellow Fever in Ghana when investigating disease.

GERMANY
**1928** Ascheim and Zondek introduce first usable pregnancy test. **1932** Anti-malarial drug, atebrin, (mepacrine) synthesised by Mietzsch, Mauss and Walter Kikuth. **1935** Domagh finds that pronotosil, a dye stuff derived from sulphanilamide, protects mice against fatal doses of streptococci.

BRITAIN
**1953** Structure of DNA discovered by Crick and Watson.

NETHERLANDS
Einthoven invents ...g galvanometer, ...practical ECG ...rocardiograph).
...Rocci invents ...gmomanometer ...asure blood ...ure.

BRITAIN
**1904** Bayliss and Starling discover chemicals stimulate secretions: theory of hormonal control of these develops.

PORTUGAL
**1935** First pre-frontal leucotomy introduced by Moniz; used to treat certain psychoses.

INDIA
**1955** Optical fibres invented by Kapany.

USA
**1903** Aeroplane invented by Wright brothers.

SWITZERLAND
**1911** Bleuler proposes the term 'schizophrenia'

USA
Inventions **1925** Frozen food process by Birds Eye. **1928** Electric razor by Schick. **1938** Xerography by Chester Carbon.

**1939-1945** Second World War. Atomic bomb invented by Frisch, Bohr and Peieris. Penicillin used to treat wound infections.
**1936-39** Spanish Civil War.
**1935-1936** Abyssinian War.

**1953** Edmund Hillary and Sherpa Tensing reach the summit of Mount Everest.

**1952** Hydrogen bomb tested.

**1950-1953** Korean War.

BRITAIN
Vacuum invented by Booth. **1912** Loss of RMS ...ic. **1912** Captain Scott's ill-fated expedition ...es South Pole. **1913** Geiger counter by Geiger.

GERMANY
**1914-1918** First World War: 'Shell-shocked' patients.

**1916** Einstein publishes General Theory of Relativity.

BRITAIN
**1922** Tutankhamun's tomb discovered. **1925/1926** Baird invents television. **1929** Decompression chamber invented by Robert H. Davis. **1935** Watson-Watt invent radar.

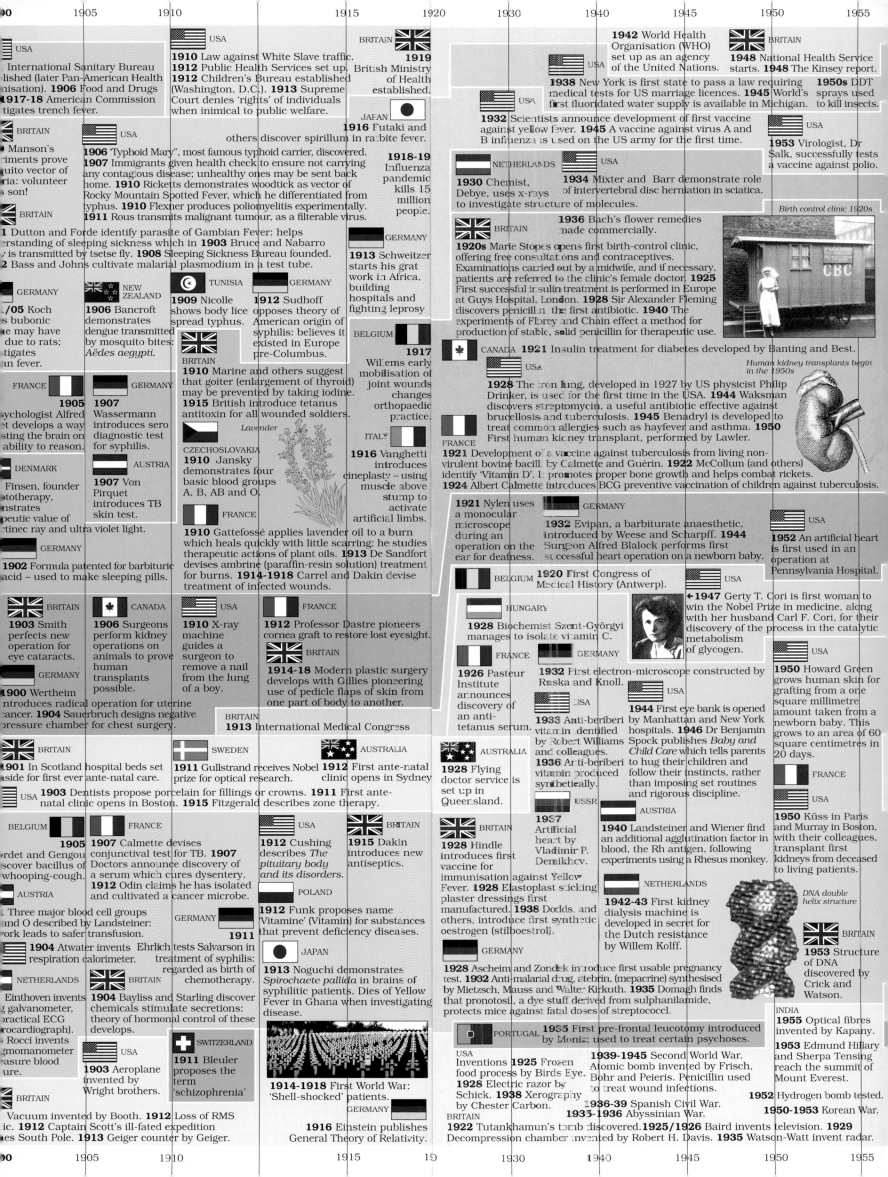

**Society**

**Public health**

AUSTRALIA

**1955** WHO (World Health Organisation) declares that, with DDT and world support, malaria may be eradicated. **1955** WHO says that atomic waste poses serious health risk. **1960s** Toxicity of DDT better understood: DDT spraying becomes less common.

**1969** WHO admits plan to eradicate malaria has failed.

**1980** WHO announces smallpox is completely eradicated. Later accidental infection at Birmingham of laboratory technician; professor commits suicide.

**1996** The world's fir[st] permitting euthana[sia] comes into force an[d] terminally ill cancer patient becomes firs[t] die under this volun[tary] euthanasia legislati[on]

SWITZERLAND

**1996** WHO set up a[n] obesity task force t[o] combat a worldwide epidemic of obesity

**Disease**

**1963** Measles vaccine introduced.

USA

**1972** Syphilis Scandal: it was revealed that the Public Health Service has been studying syphilis in black men in Macon County, Alabama for 40 years without treating them. **1981** AIDS first recognised in New York and Los Angeles. **1992** Doctors say Legionnaire's Disease can be caught via tap water as well as air-conditioning systems. **1996** Scientists believe they may have identified cause of addiction to cigarette smoking.

BRITAIN

**1990** Scientists deny BSE poses a threat but in **1991** the first woman dies of Creutzfeld Jakob's disease, the human form of 'mad cow disease'.

BRITAIN

**1991** Doctors develop a method of estimating when a patient infected with HIV may develop full-blown AIDS.

**1958** Thalidomide shown to cause birth defects.

NEW ZEALAND

**1963** Doctors give the world's first successful blood transfusion to an unborn baby.

**1960** Enders and others develop attenuated measles virus vaccine.

**Diagnosis**

USA

**Treatment**

BRITAIN

**1987** Prozac is licensed by the US Food and Drug Administration. **1988** Studies show osteopathic manipulation improves recovery time for lower back pain. **1995** In tests, a hand-held cancer 'supergun' halts tumour growth in mice. It shoots microscopic gold 'bullets', coated with genetic material, into the body. These enter the cancers and stimulate the body's immune system to fight them. **1998** Viagra, the new anti-impotence treatment, is approved by the US Food and Drugs Administration. **1999** Scientists develop technique for growing replacement bones: a woman is having her face rebuilt using bone grown on a mould attached to another part of her body.

**1996** New treatment f[or] cancer is tried: 2 childr[en] given cell transplants [of] umbilical cords of new [born] siblings – similar to us[e] of bone-marrow transp[lants]

SWEDEN

**1968** Epidural anaesthesia relieves pain of childbirth.

**WORLDWIDE** Ultrasound, endoscopy, gastrocopy and cancer x-rays all improve diagnosis and treatment procedures.

**1958** Ake Senning implants the first internal heart pacemaker.

AUSTRALIA

**1976** Shannon develops a bionic artificial arm with a strong hand grip. **1999** Doctors in Sydney succeed in combining the genetical material of two donor mothers into one egg. The technique may give a chance of motherhood to older women whose eggs are imperfect. So far, 3 boys and 2 girls have been born, using this technique.

**1997** Government announces ban on sal[e of] beef on the bone after evidence that BSE 'ma[d cow] disease' can be spread through bone marrow. A report in *Nature* mag[azine] suggests HIV virus responsible for AIDS appeared in humans in [the] in the late 1940s. The[ virus] was not identified unti[l the] 1980s, by which time [AIDS] is a worldwide epidem[ic]

USA

**1956** First successful kidney transplant was carried out between identical twins by Merrill and others. **1982** First operation to implant an artificial heart in a human being in Utah. **1992** A 35-year old man is given a baboon liver transplant by surgeons at Pittsburgh – but dies of a stroke three months later. The postmortem shows he had been infected with the AIDS virus. ↓

BRITAIN

**1967** St Christopher's Hospice in London pioneers hospice care for the terminally ill. **1989** Studies show osteopathic manipulation improves recovery time for lower back pain patients. **1995** Trials at Royal Marsden Hospital, London, show massage reduces anxiety and improves quality of life in cancer patients. **1996** WHO announces breakthrough in birth control for men: a weekly injection reduces sperm production to a negligible level. **1997** A five-day-old baby, given a new liver, is Britain's youngest transplant patient. **1998** A report in *New Scientist* states men who regularly give blood are less likely to suffer heart disease – seeming to support ancient medical practice of blood letting. The only leech farm in Britain (near Swansea) sells 20,000 each year to specialist hospitals such as burns units. **1999** Dolly the Sheep shows signs of accelerated genetic ageing, raising new fears about cloning humans. The sheep, the first mammal cloned from an adult, appears perfectly normal but on a genetic level is at least 6 years older than she should be; DNA sequences which protect the ends of chromosomes are shorter in Dolly than in a normal sheep of her age.

**1999** New immunisati[on] programme against Meningitis C announce[d]

AFRICA

**1996** 10 people die o[f] Ebola virus after eati[ng] chimpanzee in Gabon

GERMANY

**1999** Ebola: suspecte[d case] in Berlin may be 1st i[n] Europe. Scientists wo[rk] on plant from West Af[rica] which may help contro[l it]

**Surgery**

GERMANY

**1979** First human liver transplant.

**1986** Keyhole surgery develops.

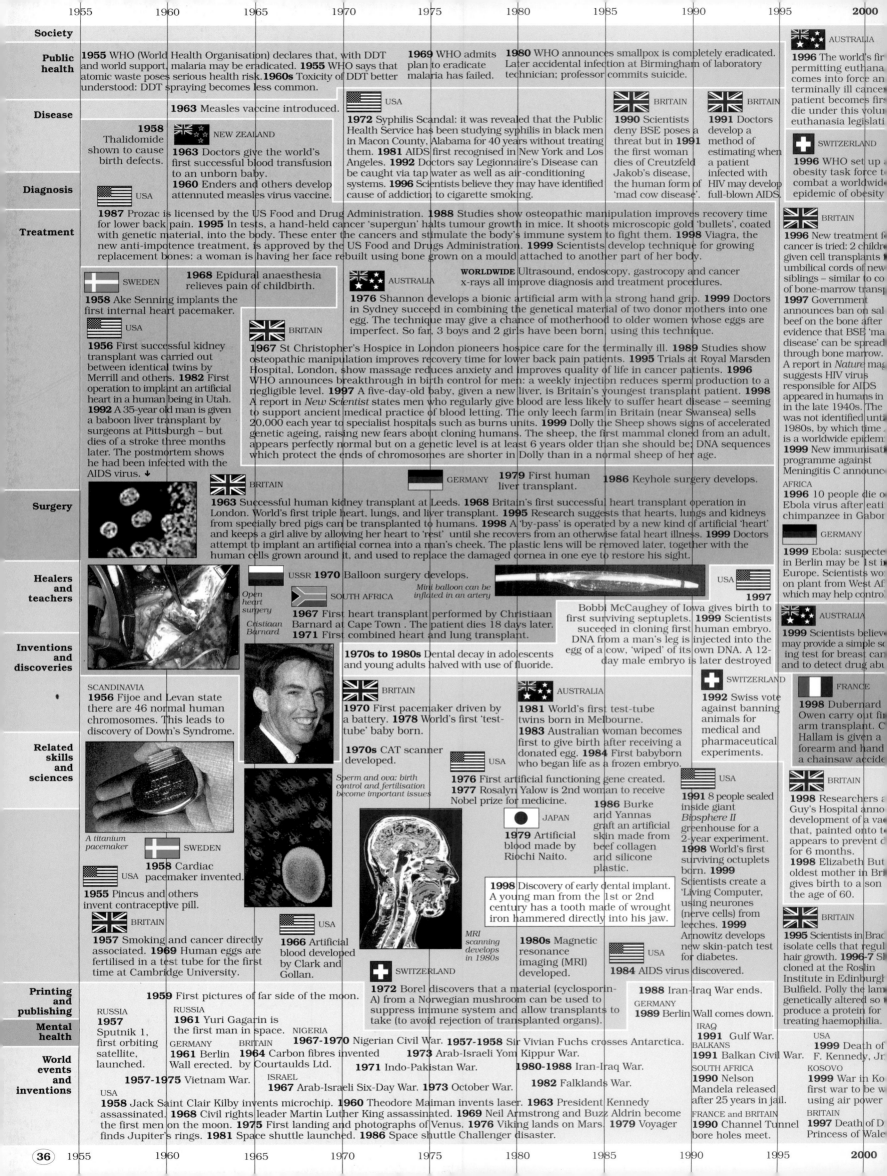

BRITAIN

**1963** Successful human kidney transplant at Leeds. **1968** Britain's first successful heart transplant operation in London. World's first triple heart, lungs, and liver transplant. **1995** Research suggests that hearts, lungs and kidneys from specially bred pigs can be transplanted to humans. **1998** A 'by-pass' is operated by a new kind of artificial 'heart' and keeps a girl alive by allowing her heart to 'rest' until she recovers from an otherwise fatal heart illness. **1999** Doctors attempt to implant an artificial cornea into a man's cheek. The plastic lens will be removed later, together with the human cells grown around it, and used to replace the damaged cornea in one eye to restore his sight.

**Healers and teachers**

USSR **1970** Balloon surgery develops.

*Mini balloon can be inflated in an artery*

USA

**1997**

*Open heart surgery*

*Cristiaan Barnard*

SOUTH AFRICA

**1967** First heart transplant performed by Christiaan Barnard at Cape Town. The patient dies 18 days later. **1971** First combined heart and lung transplant.

Bobbi McCaughey of Iowa gives birth to first surviving septuplets. **1999** Scientists succeed in cloning first human embryo. DNA from a man's leg is injected into the egg of a cow, 'wiped' of its own DNA. A 12-day male embryo is later destroyed

AUSTRALIA

**1999** Scientists believe [they] may provide a simple s[creen-]ing test for breast can[cer] and to detect drug abu[se]

**Inventions and discoveries**

**1970s to 1980s** Dental decay in adolescents and young adults halved with use of fluoride.

SWITZERLAND

**1992** Swiss vote against banning animals for medical and pharmaceutical experiments.

FRANCE

**1998** Dubernard [and] Owen carry out fir[st] arm transplant. C[live] Hallam is given a forearm and hand [after] a chainsaw accide[nt]

SCANDINAVIA

**1956** Fijoe and Levan state there are 46 normal human chromosomes. This leads to discovery of Down's Syndrome.

**Related skills and sciences**

BRITAIN

**1970** First pacemaker driven by a battery. **1978** World's first 'test-tube' baby born.

**1970s** CAT scanner developed.

AUSTRALIA

**1981** World's first test-tube twins born in Melbourne. **1983** Australian woman becomes first to give birth after receiving a donated egg. **1984** First baby born who began life as a frozen embryo.

USA

**1991** 8 people sealed inside giant *Biosphere II* greenhouse for a 2-year experiment. **1998** World's first surviving octuplets born. **1999** Scientists create a 'Living Computer', using neurones (nerve cells) from leeches. **1999** Arnowitz develops new skin-patch test for diabetes.

BRITAIN

**1998** Researchers a[t] Guy's Hospital anno[unce] development of a vac[cine] that, painted onto t[eeth] appears to prevent d[ecay] for 6 months. **1998** Elizabeth But[ler,] oldest mother in Bri[tain,] gives birth to a son [at] the age of 60.

USA

**1976** First artificial functioning gene created. **1977** Rosalyn Yalow is 2nd woman to receive Nobel prize for medicine.

*Sperm and ova: birth control and fertilisation become important issues*

JAPAN

**1979** Artificial blood made by Riochi Naito.

**1986** Burke and Yannas graft an artificial skin made from beef collagen and silicone plastic.

*A titanium pacemaker*

SWEDEN

**1958** Cardiac pacemaker invented.

USA

**1955** Pincus and others invent contraceptive pill.

BRITAIN

**1957** Smoking and cancer directly associated. **1969** Human eggs are fertilised in a test tube for the first time at Cambridge University.

USA

**1966** Artificial blood developed by Clark and Gollan.

*MRI scanning develops in 1980s*

**1998** Discovery of early dental implant. A young man from the 1st or 2nd century has a tooth made of wrought iron hammered directly into his jaw.

**1980s** Magnetic resonance imaging (MRI) developed.

USA

**1984** AIDS virus discovered.

BRITAIN

**1995** Scientists in Brad[ford] isolate cells that regul[ate] hair growth. **1996-7** Sh[eep] cloned at the Roslin Institute in Edinburg[h.] Bulfield. Polly the lam[b,] genetically altered so t[o] produce a protein for treating haemophilia.

**Printing and publishing**

**Mental health**

**World events and inventions**

**1959** First pictures of far side of the moon.

SWITZERLAND

**1972** Borel discovers that a material (cyclosporin-A) from a Norwegian mushroom can be used to suppress immune system and allow transplants to take (to avoid rejection of transplanted organs).

**1988** Iran-Iraq War ends.

GERMANY

**1989** Berlin Wall comes down.

RUSSIA
**1957** Sputnik 1, first orbiting satellite, launched.

RUSSIA
**1961** Yuri Gagarin is the first man in space.

GERMANY
**1961** Berlin Wall erected.

BRITAIN
**1964** Carbon fibres invented by Courtaulds Ltd.

NIGERIA
**1967-1970** Nigerian Civil War.

**1957-1958** Sir Vivian Fuchs crosses Antarctica.

**1973** Arab-Israeli Yom Kippur War.

**1971** Indo-Pakistan War.

**1980-1988** Iran-Iraq War.

IRAQ
**1991** Gulf War.

BALKANS
**1991** Balkan Civil War.

SOUTH AFRICA
**1990** Nelson Mandela released after 25 years in jail.

USA
**1999** Death of J[ohn] F. Kennedy, Jr.

KOSOVO
**1999** War in Ko[sovo,] first war to be w[on] using air power.

**1957-1975** Vietnam War.

ISRAEL
**1967** Arab-Israeli Six-Day War. **1973** October War.

**1982** Falklands War.

FRANCE and BRITAIN
**1990** Channel Tunnel bore holes meet.

BRITAIN
**1997** Death of D[iana,] Princess of Wale[s]

USA
**1958** Jack Saint Clair Kilby invents microchip. **1960** Theodore Maiman invents laser. **1963** President Kennedy assassinated. **1968** Civil rights leader Martin Luther King assassinated. **1969** Neil Armstrong and Buzz Aldrin become the first men on the moon. **1975** First landing and photographs of Venus. **1976** Viking lands on Mars. **1979** Voyager finds Jupiter's rings. **1981** Space shuttle launched. **1986** Space shuttle Challenger disaster.

No-one can predict the future. Advances in medicine may develop from revolutionary ideas and discoveries – as yet undreamed of – that will change the current direction of development, while many of those concepts that seem feasible now could perhaps fail the test of time.

It is evident that microsurgery and minimal access surgery, organ transplant and genetic engineering, robot engineering and single-use disposable or re-sposable instruments will influence the new surgery.

**Microsurgery** is already revolutionising the operating theatre. Surgeons view the site through a powerful electron microscope and computer controlled robotic hands are manipulated to operate the minute electronic surgical instruments.

Meanwhile surgeons can operate deep into the brain or ear with **laser surgery**. The laser beam vapourises unwanted tissues so these operations are bloodless and, as the light can be directed down tiny optical fibres, it can be used inside arteries, in the heart and on the eye.

Laser and **electrosurgery** are likely to be used in ever more sophisticated ways, with the active compo-

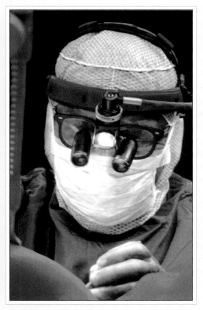

*The new face of surgery*

nents an inherent part of the surgeon's instruments. In time, even more sophisticated robotics may well mean that the surgeon operates by remote control, guiding the tools from a 'control room' by virtual reality.

Extremely fine instruments that can stitch veins, nerves and capillaries are helping to greatly improve the success rate of reconnecting **severed limbs**. When speed is of the essence, special microscopes allow several surgeons to operate at once.

**Genetic engineering** is only in its infancy. It is likely to have an enor-

mous impact on surgery and many other fields of medicine.

Of course, however much the means of diagnosis and treatment continue to improve, the actual **medical problems and disease** will not vanish. Unknown and mutated forms of disease continue to emerge and resistant strains of bacteria to appear. The spread of AIDS is likely to continue to cause concern although new ways of treating the disease are now being researched. Drug abuse remains a huge issue that may have long-term effects on our society. Meanwhile, advances in the battle against cancer, heart disease and infertility seem bound to feature in our future world.

Conventional X- rays will probably be used less and less as the latest methods of **scanning** improve and become more mobile.

The now familiar heart/lung machine and kidney dialysis machine will undoubtedly be joined by other similar devices, **machines** that can temporarily take over the functions of the different **body organs**, especially during operations, when it is important that as much of the patient's blood as possible is able to be recovered and recycled.

Current trends would suggest an increased influence of Eastern medicine, with **alternative and complementary medicine** becoming generally more acceptable – along with an holistic approach to healing.

### New ideas and developments in 1999 include the following:

### Intelligent instruments

There seems enormous scope for the future development of 'intelligent' surgical and diagnostic instruments. Already there are 'chip on a stick' endoscopes that incorporate and use a camera as part of the instrument. It is now evident that a wide variety of functions could be accommodated – these might include ultra-sound, pressure and flow – in minimally interventional devices.

Intelligent instruments will carry their own power supply and be able to communicate with other systems using links such as infra red

### 'Laboratory on a chip'

Histology, blood, gas analysis, and on-line bacteriology should soon be able to be obtained in theatre using semi-conductor technology to detect the complex metabolic materials. Meanwhile, new materials mean that instruments will become lighter and more flexible, and endoscopes should be better able to 'see' around and behind structures.

### Cancer control

A common starfish that is found in the English Channel, *Marthasterias Glacialis*, lays eggs containing a particularly high level of an enzyme (cyclin dependent kinases) that regulates cell growth. Scientists at Newcastle University, UK believe this may prove useful in controlling the growth of cancer cells.

### Testing for disease

Scientists at Dundee University, UK, may have found an alternative to blood tests or biopsies by making what they have termed a 'flapjack'! This contains a 'marker' substance which can help doctors make a diagnosis. The patient breathes into a tube after eating the 'flapjack' – and the samples can then be analysed to collect information on diseases such as AIDS, diabetes, dyspepsia and irritable bowel syndrome. This is obviously less distressing than the present means of testing available.

### Diabetic testing

A new invention by may help reduce the discomfort of testing levels of sugar in diabetic patients. At present they need to monitor their blood sugar by taking a small sample with a needle-stick test every day. A USA scientist in Florida, Jack Aronowitz, has created a new system whereby a tiny gel patch can penetrate the skin and analyse sugar levels without breaking the skin surface. Once the gel has reacted with the sugar it crosses back and reacts with the patch, changing its colour according to the level of sugar. This process takes about five minutes, after which the patch is peeled off and put under a meter that measures the subtle change in colour and provides a digital output of the blood sugar level.

### Leeches

The next generation of computers may harness living cells. USA Professor Bill Ditto and his team have succeeded in prompting nerve cells to do mathematics by taking neurones out of leeches, and 'letting them organise themselves to do computations'. Neurones (the basic communication units the brain uses) can think for themselves, respond to new situations, and learn from experience. In these latest experiments, leech nerve cells are hooked up to a computer, stimulated with electrodes to make them communicate, programmed with numbers, and then – when the cells are connected together – they will add up and produce an answer. This study of neurones and brain functions may well have implications in the medical field.

THE FUTURE

**WHAT LIES
AHEAD?**

**27 June 2000**

Scientists from six countries (USA, UK, Germany, France, China and Japan) working on the The Human Genome Project have 'cracked the code' of DNA genetics. Being able to decipher the code means they can now map almost the entire text of 3 billion molecular 'letters'. This breakthrough will have a huge impact on the future of science and medicine.

# NOBEL

## PRIZE WINNERS

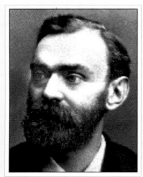

### Alfred Nobel

Swedish scientist and inventor Alfred Bernhard Nobel (1833-1896) was the founder of the Nobel Prize.

A brilliant linguist, chemist, engineer and entrepreneur, Alfred Nobel studied explosives and accrued a huge fortune from the manufacture of these, including dynamite, and from the exploitation of oil fields. In due course he established factories and laboratories in ninety different sites in twenty countries. Nobel also invented synthetic rubber and fabrics and by the time of his death had 355 patents.

From a fund established under his will, the prestigious Nobel prizes have been awarded annually since 1901, the fifth anniversary of Alfred Nobel's death.

### 1901

**Physics**      GERMANY
Wilhelm Röntgen - Discovery of X-rays.

**Chemistry**   NETHERLANDS
Jacobus Van't Hoff - Laws of chemical dynamics & osmotic pressure.

**Medicine**      GERMANY
Emil von Behring - Work on serum therapy.

### 1902

**Physics**     NETHERLANDS
Hendrik Lorentz, Pieter Zeeman - Investigation of the influence of magnetism on the phenomena of radiation.

**Chemistry**      GERMANY
Emil Fischer - Work on sugar and purine syntheses.

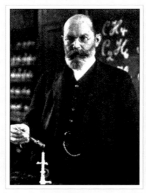

**Medicine**            UK
Sir Ronald Ross - Discovery of how malaria enters an organism.

### 1903

**Physics**          FRANCE
Antoine Henri Becquerel, Pierre Curie, Marie Curie - Joint work concerning investigations of the radiation phenomena discovered by A.H. Becquerel.

**Chemistry**      SWEDEN
Svante Arrhenius - Theory of electrolytic dissociation.

**Medicine**      DENMARK
Niels R Finsen - Treatment of skin diseases with light radiation.

### 1904

**Physics**            UK
Lord Rayleigh - Discovery of argon.

**Chemistry**            UK
Sir William Ramsay - Discovery of inert gaseous elements and determination of their places in the periodic system.

**Medicine**          RUSSIA
Ivan Pavlov - Work on the physiology of digestion.

### 1905

**Physics**          GERMANY
Philipp Lenard - Research on cathode rays.

**Medicine**          GERMANY
Robert Koch - Tuberculosis research.

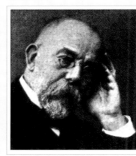

**Chemistry**          GERMANY
Adolf von Baeyer - Work on organic dyes, hydroaromatic compounds.

### 1906

**Physics**            UK
Sir Joseph Thomson - Researches into electrical conductivity of gases

**Chemistry**          FRANCE
Henri Moissan - Isolation of fluorine; introduction of Moissan furnace.

**Medicine**      ITALY SPAIN
Camillo Golgi, S. Ramón y Cajal - Work on the structure of the nervous system.

### 1907

**Physics**            USA
Albert Michelson - Spectroscopic and metrological investigations using precision optical instruments.

**Medicine**          FRANCE
Alphonse Laveran - Discovery of the role of protozoa in diseases.

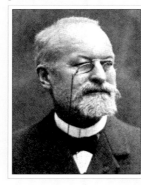

**Chemistry**          GERMANY
Eduard Buchner - Discovery of noncellular fermentation.

### 1908

**Physics**          FRANCE
Gabriel Lippmann - Photographic reproduction of colours.

**Medicine** GERMANY RUSSIA
Paul Ehrlich, Elie Metchnikoff - Work on immunity.

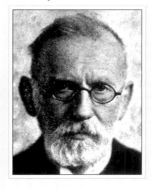

**Chemistry**            UK
Lord Rutherford - Investigations into the disintegration of elements and the chemistry of radioactive substances.

### 1909

**Physics**     ITALY GERMANY
Guglielmo Marconi, Karl Braun - Development of wireless telegraphy.

**Chemistry**          GERMANY
Wilhelm Ostwald - Pioneer work on catalysis, chemical equilibrium and reaction velocities.

**Medicine**      SWITZERLAND
Emil Kocher - Physiology, pathology and surgery of thyroid gland.

### 1910

**Physics**     NETHERLANDS
J. van der Waals - Research concerning the equation of state of gases and liquids.

**Chemistry**          GERMANY
Otto Wallach - Pioneer work in alicyclic combinations.

**Medicine**          GERMANY
Albrecht Kossel - Researches in cellular chemistry.

### 1911

**Physics**          GERMANY
Wilhelm Wien - Discoveries regarding laws governing heat radiation.

**Chemistry**          FRANCE
Marie Curie - Discovery of radium and polonium; isolation of radium.

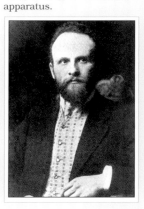

**Medicine**          SWEDEN
Allvar Gullstrand - Work on dioptrics of the eye.

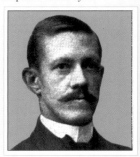

### 1912

**Physics**          SWEDEN
Nils Gustaf Dalén - Invention of automatic regulators for lighting coastal beacons and light buoys during darkness or other periods of reduced visibility.

**Chemistry**          FRANCE
Victor Grignard - Discovery of the so-called Grignard reagents.

**Chemistry**          FRANCE
Paul Sabatier - Method of hydrogeneting organic compounds in the presence of finely powdered metals.

**Medicine**          FRANCE
Alexis Carrel - Work on vascular suture; transplantation of organs and blood vessels.

**Physics**     NETHERLANDS
H. Kamerlingh Onnes - Investigation into the properties of matter at low temperatures; production of liquid helium.

### 1913

**Chemistry**   SWITZERLAND
Alfred Werner - Work on the linkage of atoms in molecules.

**Medicine**          FRANCE
Charles Richet - Work on anaphylaxis.

### 1914

**Medicine**          AUSTRIA
Robert Bárány - Physiology and pathology of vestibular apparatus.

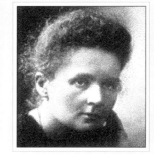

**Physics** GERMANY
Max von Laue - Discovery of diffraction of x-rays by crystals.

**Chemistry** USA
Theodore Richards - Accurate determination of the atomic weights of numerous elements.

## 1915

**Physics** UK
Sir William Bragg, Sir Lawrence Braff - Analysis of crystal structure by means of x-rays.

**Chemistry** GERMANY
Richard Willstätter - Pioneer researches on plant pigments, especially chlorophyll.

## 1917

**Physics** UK
Charles Barkla - Discovery of characteristic x-radiation of elements.

## 1918

**Physics** GERMANY
Max Planck - Discovery of the elemental quanta.

**Chemistry** GERMANY
Fritz Haber - Synthesis of ammonia from its elements.

## 1919

**Physics** GERMANY
Joahannes Stark - Discovery of the Doppler effect in canal rays and of the division of spectral lines in the electric field.

**Medicine** BELGIUM
Jules Bordet - Discoveries in regard to immunity.

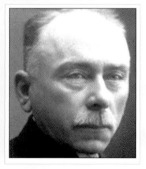

## 1920

**Physics** SWITZERLAND
Charles Guillaume - Discovery of anomalies in nickel-steel alloys.

**Chemistry** GERMANY
Walther Nernst - Work in thermochemistry.

**Medicine** DENMARK
August Krogh - Discovery of capillary motor regulating mechanism.

## 1921

**Physics** GERMANY SWITZERLAND
Albert Einstein - Services to theoretical physics, especially discovery of law of photoelectric effect.

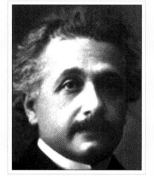

**Chemistry** UK
Frederick Soddy - Chemistry of radioactive substances; occurrence and nature of isotopes.

## 1922

**Physics** DENMARK
Niels Bohr - Investigation of atomic structure and radiation.

**Chemistry** UK
Francis Aston - Work with mass spectrograph; whole-number rule.

**Medicine** UK
Archibald V. Hill - Discovery relating to heat production in muscles.

**Medicine** GERMANY
Otto Meyerhof - Discovery of correlation between oxygen consumption and metabolism of lactic acid in muscles.

## 1923

**Physics** USA
Robert Millikan - Work on elementary electric charge and the photoelectric effect.

**Chemistry** AUSTRIA
Fritz Pregl - Method of microanalysis of organic substances.

**Medicine** CANADA UK
Sir F.G. Banting, J.J.R. Macleod - Discovery of insulin.

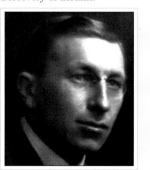

## 1924

**Physics** SWEDEN
Karl Siegbahn - Discoveries and investigations in x-ray spectroscopy.

**Medicine** NETHERLANDS
Willem Einthoven - Discovery of electrocardiogram mechanism.

## 1925

**Physics** GERMANY
James Franck, Gustav Hertz - Discovery of the laws governing the impact of an electron on an atom.

**Chemistry** AUSTRIA
Richard Zsigmondy - Elucidation of the heterogeneous nature of colloidal solutions.

## 1926

**Physics** FRANCE
Jean Baptiste Perrin - Works on discontinuous structure of matter, especially the discovery of the equilibrium of sedimentation.

**Chemistry** SWEDEN
Theodor Svedberg - Work on disperse systems.

**Medicine** DENMARK
Johannes Fibiger - Discovery of Spiroptera carcinoma.

## 1927

**Physics** USA
Arthur Holly Compton - Discovery of wave-length change in diffused x-rays.

**Physics** UK
Charles Wilson - Method of making visible the paths of electrically charged particles by vapour condensation.

**Chemistry** GERMANY
Heinrich Wieland - Researches into the constitution of bile acids.

**Medicine** AUSTRIA
J. Wagner von Jauregg - Discovery of therapeutic importance of malaria inoculation in *dementia paralytica*.

## 1928

**Physics** UK
Sir Owen Richardson - Discovery of Richardson's law (the dependency of the emission of electrons on temperature).

**Chemistry** GERMANY
Adolf Windaus - Constitution of sterols and their connection with vitamins.

**Medicine** FRANCE
Charles Nicolle - Work on typhus.

## 1929

**Physics** FRANCE
Prince Louis de Broglie - Discovery of the wave nature of electrons.

**Chemistry** UK SWEDEN
Sir Arthur Harden, H. von Euler-Chelpin - Investigations on the fermentation of sugars and the enzymes acting in this connection.

**Medicine** NETHERLANDS
Christiaan Eijkmann - Discovery of antineuritic vitamin.

**Medicine** UK
Sir F. Hopkins - Discovery of growth-stimulating vitamins.

## 1930

**Physics** INDIA
Sir C. Raman - Work on light diffusion; discovery of Raman effect.

**Chemistry** GERMANY
Hans Fischer - Hemin, chlorophyll research; synthesis of hemin.

**Medicine** USA
Karl Landsteiner - Grouping of human blood.

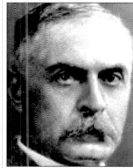

## 1931

**Chemistry** GERMANY
Karl Bosch, Friedrich Bergius - Invention and development of chemical high-pressure methods.

**Medicine** GERMANY
Otto Warburg - Discovery of nature and action of respiratory enzyme.

## 1932

**Physics** GERMANY
Werner Heisenberg - Creation of quantum mechanics.

**Chemistry** USA
Irving Langmuir - Discoveries and investigations in surface chemistry.

**Medicine** UK
Edgar D. Adrian, Sir C. Sherrington - Discovering functions of neurons.

## 1933

**Physics** UK AUSTRIA
Paul Dirac, Erwin Schrödinger - Discovery of new fruitful forms of atomic energy.

**Medicine** USA
Thomas Hunt Morgan - Heredity transmission functions of chromosomes.

## 1934

**Chemistry** USA
Harold Urey - Discovery of heavy hydrogen.

**Medicine** USA
George R. Minot, William P. Murphy, George H. Whipple - Discoveries concerning liver therapy against anaemia.

## 1935

**Physics** UK
Sir James Chadwick - Discovery of neutron.

**Chemistry** FRANCE
Frédéric Joliot, Irène Joliot-Curie - Synthesis of new radioactive elements.

**Medicine** GERMANY
Hans Spemann - Organizer effect in embryonic development.

## 1936

**Physics** AUSTRIA
Victor Hess - Discovery of cosmic radiation.

**Physics** USA
Carl Anderson - Discovery of positron.

**Chemistry** NETHERLANDS
Peter Debye - Studies of dipole moments and the diffraction of x-rays and electrons in gases.

**Medicine** UK GERMANY
Sir H.H. Dale, Otto Loewi - Discoveries relating to the chemical transmission of nerve impulses.

## 1937

**Physics** USA UK
Clinton Davisson, Sir George Thomson - Experimental discovery of the interference phenomenon in crystals irradiated by electrons.

**Chemistry** UK
Sir Walter Haworth - Research on carbohydrates and vitamic C.

**Chemistry**  SWITZERLAND
Paul Karrer -
Research on carotenoids,
flavins and vitamins.

**Medicine**  HUNGARY
Albert Szent-Györgyi -
Work on biological
combustion.

### 1938

**Physics**  ITALY
Enrico Fermi -
Disclosure of artificial
radioactive elements
produced by neutron
irradiation.

**Chemistry**  GERMANY
Richard Kuhn -
Carotenoid and vitamin
research (declined).

**Medicine**  BELGIUM
Corneille Heymans -
Discovery of role of sinus
and aortic mechanism in
respiration regulation.

### 1939

**Physics**  USA
Ernest Lawrence -
Invention of the cyclotron.

**Chemistry**  GERMANY
Adolf Butenandt -
Work on sexual hormones
(declined).

**Chemistry**  SWITZERLAND
Leopold Ruzicka -
Work on polymethylenes and
higher terpenes.

**Medicine**  GERMANY
Gerhard Domagk -
Antibacterial effect of
prontosil (declined).

### 1943

**Physics**  USA
Otto Stern -
Discovery of the magnetic
moment of the proton.

**Chemistry**  HUNGARY
George de Hevesy -
Use of isotopes as traces
in chemical research.

**Medicine**  DENMARK
Henrik Dam -
Discovery of Vitamin K.

**Medicine**  USA
Edward A. Doisy -
Discovery of chemical nature
of vitamin K.

### 1944

**Physics**  USA
Isidor Rabi -
Resonance method for
registration of magnetic
properties of atomic nuclei.

**Chemistry**  GERMANY
Otto Hahn -
Discovery of the fission of
heavy nuclei.

**Medicine**  USA
Joseph Erlanger, Herbert S.
Gasser - Researches on
differentiated function of
single nerve fibres.

### 1945

**Physics**  AUSTRIA
Wolfgang Pauli -
Discovery of the exclusion
'Pauli' principle.

**Chemistry**  FINLAND
Artturi Virtanen -
Invention of fodder
preservation method.

**Medicine**  UK AUSTRIA
Sir A. Fleming,
Ernst Boris Chain,
Lord Florey -
Discovery of penicillin and
its curative value in some
infectious diseases.

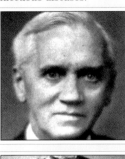

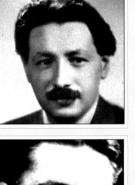

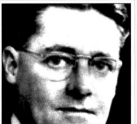

### 1946

**Physics**  USA
Percy Bridgman - Discoveries
in the domain of high-
pressure physics.

**Chemistry**  USA
James Sumner - Discovery of
enzyme crystallization.

**Chemistry**  USA
John Northrop, Wendell
Stanley - Preparation of
enzymes and virus proteins
in pure form.

**Medicine**  USA
Hermann J. Muller -
Production of mutations by
x-ray irradiation.

### 1947

**Physics**  UK
Sir Edward Appleton -
Discovery of Appleton layer
in upper atmosphere.

**Chemistry**  UK
Sir Robert Robinson -
Investigations on alkaloids
and other plant products.

**Medicine**  USA
Carl F. Cori, Gerty T. Cori -
Discovery of how glycogen is
catalytically converted.

**Medicine**  ARGENTINA
Bernardo Houssay - Pituitary
hormone function in sugar
metabolism.

### 1948

**Physics**  UK
Patrick Blackett - Discoveries
in the domain of nucleur
physics and cosmic radiation
using the Wilson cloud
chamber.

**Chemistry**  SWEDEN
Arne Tiselius - Researches
on electrophoresis and
adsorption analysis;
researches on the serum
proteins.

**Medicine**  SWITZERLAND
Paul Müller -
Properties of DDT.

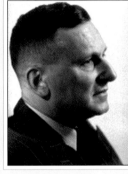

### 1949

**Physics**  JAPAN
Hideki Yukawa - Prediction
of the existence of mesons.

**Chemistry**  USA
William Giauque -
Behaviours of substances at
extremely low temperatures.

**Medicine**  SWITZERLAND
Walter Hess - Discovery of
function of middle brain.

**Medicine**  PORTUGAL
Antonio Moniz -
Therpeutic value of
leucotomy in psychoses.

### 1950

**Physics**  UK
Cecil Powell - Photographic
method of studying nuclear
process; discoveries of
mesons.

**Chemistry**  GERMANY
Otto Diels, Kurt Alder -
Discovery and development
of diene synthesis.

**Medicine**  USA
SWITZERLAND
Philip S. Hench,
Edward C. Kendall,
Tadeusz Reichstein -
Research on adrenal cortex
hormones, their structure
and biological effects.

### 1951

**Physics**  UK IRELAND
Sir John Cockcroft,
Ernest Walton -
Work on transmutation of
atomic nuclei by artificially
accelerated particles.

**Chemistry**  USA
Edwin McMillan,
Glenn Seaborg -
Discovery of and research
on transuranium elements.

### 1951

**Medicine**  SOUTH AFRICA
USA
Max Theiler -
Yellow fever discoveries.

### 1952

**Physics**  USA
Felix Bloch,
Edward Purcell -
Discovery of nuclear
magnetic resonance
in solids.

**Chemistry**  UK
Archer Martin, Richard
Synge - Method of identifying
and separating chemical
elements by
chromatography.

**Medicine**  USA
Selman Waksman -
Discovery of streptomycin.

### 1953

**Physics**  NETHERLANDS
Frits Zernike - Method of
phase-contrast microscopy.

**Chemistry**  GERMANY
Hermann Staudinger -
Work on macromolecules.

**Medicine**  GERMANY
Fritz Lipmann, Hans Krebs -
Discovery of coenzyme a
citric acid cycle in
metabolism of
carbohydrates.

### 1954

**Physics**  UK
Max Born -
Statistical studies on
wave functions.

**Physics**  GERMANY
Walther Bothe -
Invention of studies with
coincidence method.

**Chemistry**  USA
Linus Carl Pauling - Study of
the nature of the chemical
bond.

**Medicine**  USA
John Enders, Thomas Weller,
Frederick Robbins -
Cultivation of the polio-
myelitis virus in tissue
cultures.

### 1955

**Physics**  USA
Willis Lamb, Jr. -
Discoveries of magnetic
moment of electron.

**Physics**  USA
Polykark Kusch -
Measurement of magnetic
moment of electron.

**Chemistry**  USA
Vincent Du Vigneaud - First
synthesis of a polypeptide
hormone.

**Medicine**  SWEDEN
Hugo Theorell -
Nature and mode of actions
of oxidation enzymes.

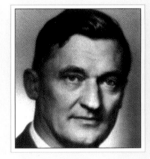

### 1956

**Physics**  USA
William Shockely, John
Bardeen, Walter Brattain -
Investigations on
semiconductors and
discovery of the
transistor effect.

**Chemistry**  USSR UK
Nikolai Semenov,
Sir Cyril Hinshelwood -
Work on the kinetics of
chemical reactions.

**Medicine**  USA GERMANY
André Cournand, Dickinson
Richards Jr., Werner
Forssmann - Discoveries
concerning heart
catheterization and
circulatatory changes.

### 1957

**Physics**  CHINA
Tsung-Dao Lee,
Chen Ning Yang -
Discovery of violations of the
principle of parity (space
reflection symmetry).

**Chemistry**  UK
Sir Alexander Todd - Work
on nucleotides and
nucleotide coenzymes.

**Medicine** ITALY
Daniel Bovet - Production of synthetic curare.

## 1958

**Physics** USSR
Pavel Cherenkov, Ilya Frank, Igor Tamm - Discovery and interpretation of the Cerekov effect (emission of light waves by electrically charged particles moving faster than light).

**Chemistry** UK
Frederick Sanger - Determination of structure of insulin molecule.

**Medicine** USA
George Beadle, Edward Tatum, Joshua Lederberg - Genetic regulation of chemical processes; genetic recombination; bacterial genetics.

## 1959

**Physics** USA
Emilio Segrè, Owen Chamberlain - Confirmation of the existence of the anti-proton.

**Chemistry** CZECHOSLOVAKIA
Jaroslav Heyrovsky - Discovery and development of polargraphy.

**Medicine** USA
Severo Ochoa, Arthur Kornberg - Work on producing nucleic acids artificially.

## 1960

**Physics** USA
Donald Glaser - Development of the bubble chamber.

**Chemistry** USA
Williard Libby - Development of radiocarbon dating.

**Medicine** AUSTRALIA UK
Sir Macfarlane Burnet, Peter Medawar - Acquired immunity to tissue transplants.

## 1961

**Medicine** HUNGARY
Georg von Békésy - Functions of the inner ear.

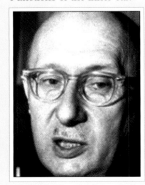

**Physics** USA
Robert Hofstadter - Determination of shape and size of atomic nucleons.

**Physics** GERMANY
Rudolf Mössbauer - Discovery of the 'Mossbauer effect'.

**Chemistry** USA
Melvin Calvin - Study of chemical steps that take place during photosynthesis.

## 1962

**Physics** USSR
Lev D. Landau - Contributions to the understanding of condensed states of matter (superfluidity in liquid helium).

**Chemistry** UK
John C. Kendrew, Max F. Perutz - Determination of the structure of hemoproteins.

**Medicine** UK USA
Francis Crick, Maurice Wilkins, James Watson - Discoveries concerning the molecular structure of deoxyribonucleic acid (DNA).

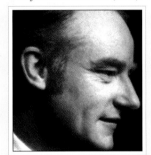

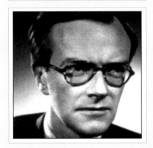

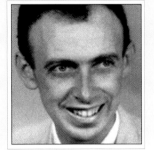

## 1963

**Physics** GERMANY USA
J. Hans D. Jensen, Maria Goeppert Mayer - Development of shell model theory of the structure of atomic nuclei.

**Physics** USA
Eugene Paul Wigner - Principles governing mechanics and interaction of protons and neutrons in the atomic nucleus.

**Chemistry** ITALY GERMANY
Giulio Natta, Karl Ziegler - Structure and synthesis of polymers in the field of plastics.

**Medicine** UK AUSTRALIA
Alan Hodgkin, Andrew Huxley, Sir John Eccles - Study of the transmission of impulses along a nerve fibre.

## 1964

**Physics** USA USSR
Charles H. Townes, Niolai G. Basov, Aleksandr M. Prokhorov - Work in quantum electronics leading to construction of instruments based on maser-laser principles.

**Chemistry** UK
Dorothy M.C. Hodgkin - Determining the structure of biochemical compounds essential in combating pernicious anemia.

**Medicine** GERMANY
Konrad Bloch, Feodor Lynen - Discoveries concerning cholesterol and fatty acid metabolism.

## 1965

**Medicine** FRANCE
François Jacob, André Lwoff, Jacques Monod - Discoveries concerning regulatory activities of body cells.

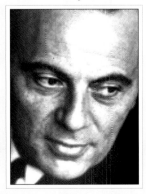

**Physics** USA JAPAN
Julian S. Schwinger, Richard P. Feynman, Shin'ichirö Tomonaga - Basic principles of quantum electrodynamics.

**Chemistry** USA
Robert B. Woodward - Synthesis of sterols, cholorophyll and other substances once thought to be produced only by living things.

## 1966

**Physics** FRANCE
Alfred Kastler - Discovery/development of optical methods for studying Hertzian resonances in atoms.

**Chemistry** USA
Robert S. Mulliken - Work concerning chemical bonds and the electronic structure of molecules by the molecular orbital method.

**Medicine** USA
Charles Huggins, Francis Peyton Rous - Research on causes and treatment of cancer.

## 1967

**Physics** USA
Hans A. Bethe - Discoveries concerning the energy production of stars.

**Chemistry** GERMANY UK
Manfreed Eigen, Ronald G.W. Norrish, George Porter - Studies of extremely fast chemical reactions.

**Medicine** SWEDEN USA
Ragnar Granit, Haldan Hartline, George Wald - Discoveries about chemical and physiological visual processes in the eye.

## 1968

**Physics** USA
Luis W. Alvarez - Work with elementary particles, including the discovery of resonance states.

**Chemistry** USA
Lars Onsager - Contributions to the theory of the thermodynamics of irreversible processes.

**Medicine** USA
Robert Holley, Har Gobind Khorana, Marshall Nirenberg - Deciphering of the genetic code.

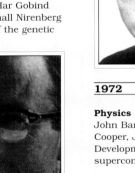

## 1969

**Physics** USA
Murray Gell-Mann - Discoveries re. classification of elementary particles and their interactions.

**Chemistry** UK NORWAY
Derek H.R. Barton, Odd Hassel - Work in determining actual three-dimensional shape of certain organic compounds.

**Medicine** USA
Max Delbrück, A.D. Hershey, Salvadore Luria - Research and discoveries concerning viruses and viral diseases.

## 1970

**Physics** SWEDEN FRANCE
Hannes Alfvén, Louis Néel - Work in magnethodhydrodynamics and in antiferromagetism and ferrimagnetism.

**Chemistry** ARGENTINA
Luis F. Leloir - Discovery of sugar nucleotides and their role in the biosynthesis of carbohydrates.

**Medicine** UK SWEDEN USA
Sir Bernard Katz, Ulf von Euler, Julius Axelrod - Discoveries concerning the chemistry of nerve transmission.

## 1971

**Physics** UK
Dennis Gabor - Invention of holography.

**Chemistry** CANADA
Gerhard Herzberg - Research in the structure of molecules.

**Medicine** USA
Earl Sutherland Jr. - Action of hormones.

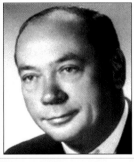

## 1972

**Physics** USA
John Bardeen, Leon N. Cooper, John R. Schrieffer - Development of the theory of superconductivity.

**Chemistry** USA
Christian B. Anfinsen, Stanford Moore, William H. Stein - Fundamental contributions to enzyme chemistry.

**Medicine** UK USA
Rodney Porter, Gerald Edelman - Research on the chemical structure of antibodies.

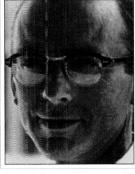

## 1973

**Physics**  JAPAN USA UK
Leo Esaki, Ivar Giaever, Brian D. Josephson - Tunnelling in semiconductors and superconductors.

**Chemistry**  GERMANY UK
Ernst Fischer, Geoffrey Wilkinson - Organometallic chemistry.

**Medicine**  GERMANY AUSTRIA UK
Karl von Frisch, Konrad Lorenz, Nikolaas Tinbergen - Discoveries in animal behaviour patterns.

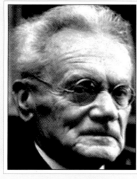

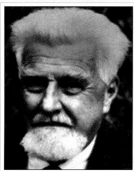

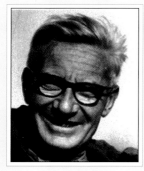

## 1974

**Physics**  UK
Sir Martin Ryle, Antony Hewish - Work in radio astronomy.

**Chemistry**  USA
Paul J. Flory - Studies of long-chain molecules.

**Medicine**  BELGIUM ROMANIA/USA
Albert Claude, Christian de Duve, George Palade - Research on structural and functional organization of cells.

## 1975

**Physics**  DENMARK USA
Aage N. Bohr, Ben R. Mottelson, L. James Rainwater - Work on the atomic nucleus.

**Chemistry**  UK SWITZERLAND
John W. Cornforth, Vladimir Prelog - Work in stereochemistry.

**Medicine**  USA ITALY
David Baltimore, Howard Temin, Renato Dulbecco - Interaction between tumour viruses and the genetic material of the cell.

## 1976

**Physics**  USA
Burton Richter, Samuel C.C. Ting - Discovery of new class of elementary particles (psi, or J).

**Chemistry**  USA
William N. Lipscomb - Structure of boranes.

**Medicine**  USA
B.S. Blumberg, D.G. Gajdusek - Studies of origin and spread of infectious diseases.

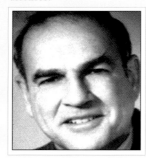

## 1977

**Physics**  USA UK
Philip W. Anderson, John H. Van Vleck, Sir Nevill F. Mott - Contributions to understanding of the behaviour of electrons in magnetic, noncrystalline solids.

**Chemistry**  BELGIUM
Ilya Prigogine - Widening the scope of thermodynamics.

**Medicine**  USA
Rosalyn Yalow - Development of radio-immunoassay.

**Medicine**  USA
R. Guillemin, A. Schally - Research on pituitary hormones.

## 1978

**Physics**  USSR
Pyotr L. Kapitsa - Invention and application of helium liquefier.

**Physics**  USA

Arno A. Penzias, Robert W. Wilson - Discovery of cosmic microwave background radiation, providing support for the big-bang theory.

**Chemistry**  UK
Peter D. Mitchell - Formulation of a theory of energy transfer processes in biological systems.

**Medicine**  SWITZERLAND USA
W. Arber, D. Nathans, H. Smith - Discovery and application of enzymes that fragment deoxyribonucleic acids.

## 1979

**Physics**  USA PAKISTAN
Sheldon Glashow, Steven Weinberg Abdus Salam - Establishment of analogy between electromagnetism and the 'weak' interactions of subatomic particles.

**Chemistry**  USA GERMANY
Herbert C. Brown, Georg Wittig - Introduction of compounds of boron and phosphorus in the synthesis of organic substances.

**Medicine**  UK USA
Godfrey Newbold Hounsfield, Allan Mcleod Cormack - Development of the CAT scan, a radiographic diagnostic technique.

## 1980

**Physics**  USA
James W. Cronin, Val Logsdon Fitch - Demonstration of simultaneous violation of both charge-conjugation and parity-inversion symmetries.

**Chemistry**  USA
Paul Berg - First preparation of a hybrid DNA.

**Chemistry**  USA UK
Walter Gilbert, Frederick Sanger - Development of chemical and biological analyses of DNA structure.

**Medicine**  USA FRANCE VENEZUELA
George Snell, Jean Dausset, Barui Benacerraf - Investigations of genetic control of the response of the immunological system to foreign substances.

## 1981

**Physics**  SWEDEN
Kai M. Siegbahn - Electron spectroscopy for chemical analysis.

**Physics**  USA
Nicolaas Bloembergen, Arthur L. Schawlow - Applications of lasers in spectroscopy.

**Chemistry**  JAPAN USA
Kenichi Fukui, Roald Hoffmann - Orbital symmetry of chemical reactions.

**Medicine**  USA
Roger Sperry - Functions of the cerebral hemispheres.

**Medicine**  USA SWEDEN
David Hubel, Torsten Wiesel - Processing of visual information by the brain.

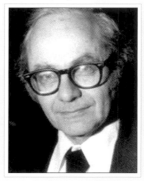

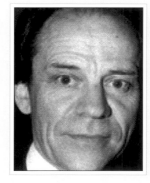

## 1982

**Physics**  USA
Kenneth G. Wilson - Analysis of continuous phase transition.

**Chemistry**  UK
Aaron Klug - Determination of structure of biological substances.

**Medicine**  SWEDEN UK
Sune K. Bergström, Bengt I. Samuelsson, John R. Vane - Biochemistry and physiology of prostaglandins.

## 1983

**Physics**  USA
Subrahmanyan Chandrasekhar, William A. Fowler - Contributions to understanding of the evolution and devolution of stars.

**Chemistry**  USA
Henry Taube - Study of electron transfer reactions.

**Physics**  USA
Barbara McClintock - Discovery of mobile plant genes which affect heredity.

## 1984

**Physics**  ITALY NETHERLANDS
Carlo Rubbia, Simon van der Meer - Discovery of subatomic particles W and Z, which supports the electroweak theory.

**Chemistry**  USA
Robert Bruce Merrifield - Development of a method of polypeptide synthesis.

**Medicine**  DENMARK GERMANY ARGENTINA/UK
Niels K. Jerne, George Köhler, Cesar Milstein - Theory and development of a technique for producing monoclonal antibodies.

## 1985

**Physics**  GERMANY
Klaus von Klitzing - Discovery of the quantized Hall effect, permitting exact measurements of electrical resistance.

**Chemistry**  USA
Herbert Hauptman, Jerome Karle - Development of way to map chemical structures of small molecules.

**Medicine**  USA
Michael Brown, Joseph Goldstein - Discovery of cell receptors relating to cholesterol metabolism.

## 1986

**Physics**  GERMANY SWITZERLAND
Ernst Ruska, Gerd Binnig, Heinrich Rohrer - Development of special electron microscopes.

**Chemistry**  USA CANADA
Dudley R. Herschbach, Yuan Lee, John Polanyi - Development of methods for analyzing basic chemical reactions.

**Medicine**  USA
Stanley Cohen, Rita Levi-Montalcini - Discovery of chemical agents that help regulate the growth of cells.

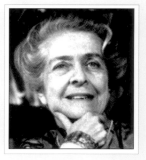

Note: The "Medicine SWITZERLAND USA" entry for W. Arber, D. Nathans, H. Smith belongs to 1978.

## 1987

**Physics**  SWITZERLAND GERMANY
Georg Bednorz,
Karl Alax Müller -
Discovery of new super
conducting materials.

**Chemistry**  USA FRANCE
Donald J. Cram, Charles J.
Pedersen, Jean-Marie Lehn -
Development of molecules
that can link with other
molecules.

**Medicine**  JAPAN
Susumu Tonegawa - Study
of genetic aspects of
antibodies.

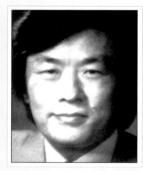

## 1988

**Physics**  USA
Leon Lederman, Melvin
Schwartz, Jack Steinberger -
Research in subatomic
particles.

**Chemistry**  GERMANY
Johann Deisenhofer, Robert
Huber, Hartmut Michel -
Discovery of structure of
proteins needed in
photosynthesis.

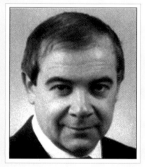

**Medicine**  UK USA
James Black, Gertrude
Elion, George Hitchings -
Development of new
classes of drugs for
combating disease.

## 1989

**Physics**  USA
Norman F. Ramsey -
Development of the atomic
clock.

**Physics**  USA GERMANY
Hans G. Dehmelt, Wolfgang
Paul - Development of
methods to isolate atoms
and subatomic particles
for study.

**Chemistry**  CANADA USA
Sidney Altman,
Thomas R. Cech -
Discovery of certain basic
properties of RNA.

**Medicine**  USA
J. Michael Bishop,
Harold E. Varmus -
Study of cancer-causing
genes called oncogenes.

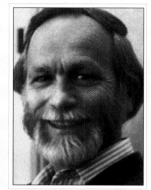

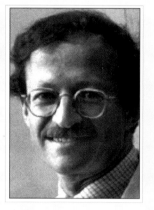

## 1990

**Medicine**  US
Joseph E. Murray,
E. Donnall Thomas -
Development of kidney and
bone-marrow transplants.

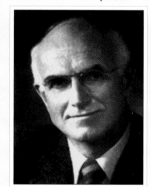

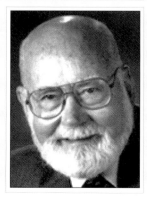

**Physics**  USA CANADA
Jerome I. Friedman,
Henry W. Kendall,
Richard E. Taylor -
Discovery of atomic quarks.

**Chemistry**  USA
Elias James Corey -
Development of 'retrosynthetic
analysis' for synthesis of
complex molecules.

## 1991

**Physics**  FRANCE
Pierre-Gilles de Gennes -
Discovery of general rules for
behaviour of molecules.

**Chemistry**  SWITZERLAND
Richard R. Ernst -
Improvements in nuclear
magnetic resonance
spectroscopy.

**Medicine**  GERMANY
Erwin Neher,
Bert Sakmann -
Discovery of how cells
communicate, as related
to diseases.

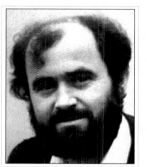

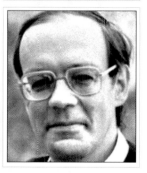

## 1992

**Physics**  FRANCE
Georges Charpak - Inventor
of detector that traces
subatomic particles.

**Chemistry**  USA
Rudolph A. Marcus -
Explanation of how electrons
transfer between molecules.

**Medicine**  US
Edmond H. Fischer, Edwin
G. Krebs - Discovery of class
of enzymes called protein
kinases.

## 1993

**Physics**  USA
Russell A. Hulse,
Joseph H. Taylor, Jr. -
Identifying binary pulsars.

**Chemistry**  USA CANADA
Kary B. Mullis,
Michael Smith -
Inventors of techniques for
gene study and
manipulation.

**Medicine**  UK US
Richard J. Roberts,
Phillip A. Sharp -
Discovery of 'split', or
interrupted, genetic
structure.

## 1994

**Physics**  CANADA USA
Bertram N. Brockhouse,
Clifford G. Shull -
Development of neutron-
scattering techniques

**Chemistry**  USA
George A. Olah -
Development of techniques
to study hydrocarbon
molecules.

**Medicine**  US
Alfred G. Gilman, Martin
Rodbell - Discovery of cell
signallers called G-proteins.

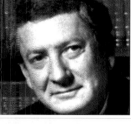

## 1995

**Physics**  USA
Martin L. Perl -
Discovery of the tau lepton.

**Physics**  USA
Frederick Reines -
Detection of the neutrino.

**Chemistry**  NETHERLANDS MEXICO USA
Paul Crutzen, Mario Molina,
F. Sherwood Rowland -
Work in atmospheric
chemistry, particularly
concerning the formation
and decomposition of ozone.

**Medicine**  USA GERMANY
Edward B. Lewis, Christiane
Nüsslein-Volhard, Eric F.
Wieschaus - Discoveries
concerning the genetic
control of early embryonic
development.

## 1996

**Physics**  USA
David M. Lee, Douglas D.
Osheroff, Robert C.
Richardson - Discovery of
superfluidity in helium-3.

**Chemistry**  USA UK
Robert F. Curl, Jr.,
Sir Harold W. Kroto,
Richard E. Smalley -
Discovery of fullerenes.

**Medicine**  AUSTRALIA SWITZERLAND
Peter C. Doherty,
Rolf M. Zinkernagel -
Discoveries concerning
the specificity of the cell
mediated immune defence.

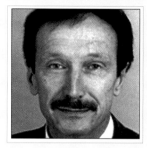

## 1997

**Physics**  USA FRANCE
Steven Chu, Claude Cohen-
Tannoudji, William D.
Phillips - Development of
methods to cool and trap
atoms with laser light.

**Chemistry**  USA UK
Paul D. Boyer, John E.
Walker - Elucidation of the
enzymatic mechanism
underlying the synthesis of
adenosine triphosphate (ATP).

**Chemistry**  DENMARK
Jens C. Skou - Discovery of
an ion-transporting enzyme,
NA+,K+-ATPase.

**Medicine**  USA
Stanley B. Prusiner -
Discovery of Prions – a new
biological principle of
infection.

## 1998

**Physics**  USA
Robert B. Laughlin, Horst L.
Störmer, Daniel C. Tsui -
Discovery of a new form
of quantum fluid with
fractionally charged
excitations.

**Chemistry**  USA
Walter Kohn - Development
of the density-functional
theory.

**Chemistry**  USA
John A. Pople - Development
of computational methods in
quantum chemistry.

**Medicine**  USA
Robert F. Furchgott, Louis J.
Ignarro, Ferid Murad -
Discoveries concerning nitric
oxide as a signalling
molecule in the
cardiovascular system.

# WOMEN

**THEIR ROLE AS DOCTORS**

*Dr Elizabeth Blackwell was the first non-cross dressing woman to attain an MD in the USA and become a doctor in 1849. She was accepted on the UK Medical Register in 1859*

Women have always been carers of the sick – and in ancient civilisations, such as Ancient Egypt and Babylonia, sometimes became skilful practitioners, especially in midwifery but also in the dressing of wounds and nursing the sick.

In the later medieval period, nuns were strongly committed to caring for the sick, while ladies of the manor developed great knowledge of herbs and other treatments.

Wise women who understood herbal remedies became a part of every community.

It was as science and formal training developed that women were allowed fewer opportunities in the medical field – except perhaps in Italy where their medical education was permitted and some women held prestigious university chairs.

## 18th and 19th centuries

In the eighteenth century Western world, it was generally believed that any intellectual activity diverted women's energies from their reproductive system and was bad for them: any attempt to pursue an academic profession was regarded with great suspicion and prejudice.

By the nineteenth century women had been thoroughly subjugated so far as the medical profession was concerned – with, as ever, the notable exceptions of midwifery and nursing. Women had always continued to be involved in obstetrics as midwifery was considered a female domain and so given scant credence as a proper science, while nursing, of course, had always been a female occupation. By 1860 Florence Nightingale had, following her great reforms in the care of the wounded and sick soldiers during the Crimean War, opened her training school for nurses at St Thomas's Hospital in London and had established nursing as a far more respectable and better organised profession. (See also the information on Florence Nightingale under the flap of the nineteenth-century section of the chart.)

However, while women could continue to demonstrate their value in certain medical areas, the idea of their becoming doctors was seen by most of the nineteenth-century establishment as ridiculous. Despite this opposition, some determined women began to prove their worth and eventually the first female doctors fought their way through repeated rejection and obstacles to achieve the necessary qualifications and grudging acceptance.

### James Barry (1797-1865)

It is believed that the Inspector General of the British Army in 1858, James Barry, who had a highly successful career in surgery for some fifty years was, in fact, a woman in disguise. Her real sex was discovered only during the autopsy that followed her death.

Her height and stature, clean-shaven face and high-pitched squeaky voice might have given her colleagues some cause for doubt but it seems that her skilled marksmanship and an aggressive attitude sufficed to ward off any suspicion.

To avoid embarrassment, the war department and medical association arranged for James Barry to be buried as a man!

### Harriot Hunt (1805-75)

In America, there was just as much opposition to women training as doctors as in Europe.

In Boston, Harriot Hunt was rejected by her fellow students after the dean there had granted her admission to Harvard Medical School – so she was forced to leave. However, she was still determined to find an entry into the medical field somehow and managed to obtained an MD degree at Syracuse as a homeopathic physician.

While not able to qualify as a fully-fledged doctor, in due course she became a professor of midwifery and of diseases of women and children at Rochester College, USA.

### Elizabeth Blackwell (1821-1910)

Elizabeth Blackwell had enormous difficulty in breaking through the wall of prejudice and resistance to women as physicians but eventually her determination and sheer hard work enabled her to achieve her ambitions. She became the first woman to be entered onto the British Medical Register as a qualified doctor.

Elizabeth Blackwell was born in England but brought up in the USA. She supported herself by teaching while she studied science in order to qualify for her entrance into college.

The Geneva College of Medicine in New York eventually admitted her. The dean agreed to accept her only if his students voted unanimously in her favour – but was very surprised when they did – it is believed this may have been as an act of capriciousness, a 'prank' to aggravate the dean. It is unlikely in the climate of the time that the male students *en masse* were seriously trying to break down the conventions of the day!

Elizabeth Blackwell proved an excellent student who gained top marks throughout the course and attained her degree in 1849.

There was still much opposition to a woman actually working in the profession but in the June of 1849, Elizabeth Blackwell began studying obstetrics in Paris, eventually went on to open a clinic for poor women and children in New York, and in 1874 she was appointed the Professor of Gynaecology at London School of Medicine for Women.

In 1860 the rules changed! Only those who had studied in British universities were allowed to register as doctors in Great Britain. In effect this excluded women doctors in the UK as no British university then allowed women to study medicine.

### Elizabeth Garrett Anderson (1836-1917)

An intelligent and well-educated young lady from a wealthy established family, Elizabeth Garrett was strongly committed to the fight for women's rights. She became involved in the Society for the Employment of Women and *The English Women's Journal* in the 1860s. It was a meeting with Elizabeth Blackwell (who wrote an article about the struggle ahead for women wishing to become physicians for *The English Women's Journal* in 1860) that inspired Elizabeth Garrett to try to become a doctor.

She worked as a student nurse at the Middlesex Hospital but was asked to leave when it was discovered that she had been unofficially attending lectures given to the medical students. Regarded as an 'impostor', she was ordered to leave.

Undeterred, she carried on studying privately with professors at both St Andrews and Edinburgh Universities and eventually became the first woman licentiate of the Society of Apothecaries in 1870 – and hence an official physician.

Elizabeth Garrett went on to run a dispensary for women and children in Marylebone and, after working with suffragettes, studied in Paris, where she finally became a Doctor of Medicine in 1870, the first British woman to achieve an MD degree.

She married and became Elizabeth Garrett Anderson, in time the mother of two girls – but still continued her work for women's causes, becoming Dean of the London School of Medicine for Women in 1883 – a post she held for twenty years.

The courage and determination of these first two women doctors 'paved the way' for others to follow and for colleges to permit them to pursue their studies, despite fierce opposition and, literally, mud-slinging: male students hurled insults and mud at women who had had to force their way through an angry mob to attend an anatomy examination in Edinburgh in 1870.

### The effect of the Great War

As in many other erstwhile male-dominated provinces, women's work at home and abroad during the First World War proved their value in the medical field, changed attitudes and greatly helped to promote their acceptance as doctors.

| Year qualifying | Women | Men |
|---|---|---|
| 1917 | 78 | 539 |
| 1918 | 68 | 341 |
| 1919 | 99 | 175 |
| 1920- | 210 | 374 |
| 1921 | 602 | 325 |

By 1985 some 5,476 women were acting as general practitioners in Britain and 20,714 men but while it is remains a male-dominated profession, the figures continue to improve.

Female hospital medical consultants rose to 21% in the UK and by 1998, 33% of general practitioners are women.

### Milestones in the UK

**1859** Elizabeth Blackwell admitted to the UK Medical Register with an American MD (Doctor of Medicine) but foreign medical degrees are subsequently disallowed.

**1865** Elizabeth Garrett obtains Licentiate of the Society of Apothecaries (who then close the loophole).

**1870** Edinburgh medical students riot against the proposed admission of women.

**1874** Founding of the London School of Medicine for Women by Sophia Jex-Blake. Although women achieve the necessary results in examinations and equal their male equivalents, they are awarded only Certificates of Proficiency, not MD degrees.

**1876** Russell Gurney's Enabling Act permits the medical licensing bodies to admit women who fulfil their requirements. Now, not only can universities can award women full medical degrees, but they can also be accepted onto the Medical Register as qualified doctors

**1877** Royal Free Hospital admits women medical students to clinical training.

**1879** Sophia Jex-Blake attempts to establish college for medical women in Edinburgh.

**1880** London Association of Medical Women established

**1880** London University recognises London School of Medicine for Women for degree purposes

**1880** 20 women on the Medical Register.

**1885** Scottish medical corporations open to women.

**1891** 101 women doctors in practice in UK.

**1892** British Medical Association admits women doctors.

**1895** Louisa Aldrich-Blake first woman to become Master of Surgery (London)

**1909** The Conjoint Examining Board recognises the London School of Medicine for Women, as well as the Royal Free, and Edinburgh Medical School for Women.

**1911** Miss E Davies-Colley becomes first female Fellow of the Royal College of Surgeons.

**1914** Outbreak of First World War: War Office initially rejects offers of service by women doctors. Their services are, however, welcomed by other allied powers.

**1916** Several London medical schools previously closed to women open their doors because of the unprecedented military and civil requirements for doctors.

**1918** 1,200 medical women practising in the UK.

**1929** First attempt to nominate a woman doctor (Christine Murrell) to the General Medical Council fails.

**1930** Medical woman appointed as Commissioner of the Board of Control.

**1930** Woman appointed Chief Medical Officer of Health of a London Borough and another as a Regional Medical Officer under NHI Acts.

**1930** A number of hospitals finally admit women to honorary staff.

**1930** The London County Council decides that from now on all medical appointments under their control – following a new Local Government Act – should be open both to men and to women.

**1933** Christine Murrell elected to the GMC but dies before she can take up her place.

**1934** Dr Helen Mackay first woman to be elected to the Fellowship of the Royal College of Physicians.

**1939** War Office agrees to appoint medical women with the same pay and allowances as medical men, and with 'relative rank' though not commissions.

**1944** About 7,200 women now on Medical Register.

**1946** National Health Service Act passed.

**1946** Women members appointed to BMA (British Medical Association) Council

**1947** All UK medical schools finally accept women.

**1948** National Health Service comes into operation.

**1949** All medical schools opened to women but a quota system (usually around 20%) continues to operate.

**1949** Medical women finally admitted to the Royal Army Medical Corps and Royal Air Force Medical Corps on short-term commissions on the same terms as men.

**1949** Professor (Later Dame) Hilda Lloyd elected President of the Royal College of Obstetricians and Gynaecologists (first woman president of a Royal College)

**1949** Professor Mary F. Lucas first woman elected President of the Anatomical Society of Great Britain and Ireland.

**1956** Dr Janet Aitken elected to the General Medical Council and first woman to take her seat.

**1956** Dr Katharine Lloyd-Williams

first woman Dean of Medical Faculty of London University.

**1956** Election of women member's representative on BMA (British Medical Association) Council

**1962** Dr Albertine Winner first woman appointed Deputy Chief Medical Officer of the Ministry of Health.

**1964** Dr Annis Gillie elected President of the College of General Practitioners.

**1965** Miss Margaret Snelling becomes first woman President of the British Institute of Radiology

**1965** Dr Albertine Winner first woman doctor appointed Honorary Physician to the Queen.

**1969** Department of Health recognises the need of married medical women for flexible postgraduate training or retraining opportunities.

**1970** Number of women on Medical Register: 23,670.

**1979** Dame Josephine Barnes becomes first woman President of the British Medical Association.

**1988** Publication of Isobel Allen's survey of doctors and their careers, *Any Room at the Top?*

**1989** Professor Margaret Turner-Warwick becomes first female President of the Royal College of Physicians.

**1990** Publication of Isobel Allen's survey *Part-time Working in General Practice.*

**1990** Dr Deidre Hine becomes first female Chief Medical Officer at the Welsh Office.

**1990** 44,000 women doctors on Medical Register (nearly 30% of total).

**1990** Proportion of women entering medical schools reaches 52%

**1993** Averil Mansfield becomes the first woman Professor of Surgery in Great Britain.

### Milestones in other countries

**1850 USA** Philadelphian Women's College of Medicine established.

**1865 Switzerland** Universities accept women students

**1869 France** Women are accepted to study medicine

**1869 Germany** Women are accepted to study medicine

**1870 Sweden** Women accepted to study medicine

**1871 Netherlands** Universities accept female medical students.

**1872 Russia** St Petersburg accepts women wanting to study to become doctors.

**1876 Ireland** The Dublin College of Physicians licenses women with existing continental degrees.

**1941 India** Indian Medical Service invites medical women to apply for temporary commissions.

**1947 USA/Czechoslovakia** Dr Gerli T. Cori – first woman to win Nobel Prize in medicine/physiology.

**1977 USA** Dr Rosalyn Yalow – second woman to win Nobel Prize in medicine.

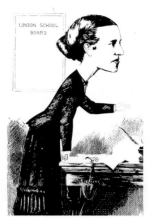

*Dr Elizabeth Garrett Anderson – a caricature*

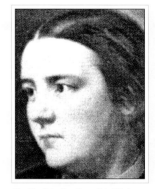

*Dr Sophia Louisa Jex Blake*

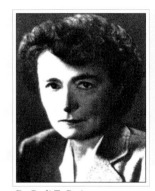

*Dr Gerli T. Cori*

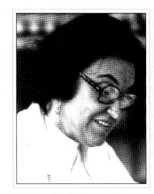

*Dr Rosalyn Yalow*

# COUNTRIES

## BRIEF SELECTION OF EVENTS

These facts extracted from the **Timechart** are, for reasons of space, necessarily limited, especially in recent decades when there have been so many developments. While they cannot, therefore, reflect the entire medical history of any nation, it is hoped they will act as a useful source of data.

### ANCIENT ASSYRIANS & BABYLONIANS

**B.C.**

**2000** Used distillation, 'essences' of cedar & volatile oils

**1900-1800** Assyrians & Babylonians see liver as seat of life • custom to lay the sick in street so that passers by can offer advice. Herodotus says every Babylonian was an amateur physician!

**1948-05** Earliest known regulations of medical practice, Code of Hammurabi: includes laws relating to medical practice

### ANCIENT CHINESE SKILLS

**B.C.**

**3494** Legendary emperor Shen Nong discovers herbal medicine

**3000-2700** Stone acupuncture needles used to treat pain

**2,698-2,598** Huang-ti's *Nei Ching*, medical compendium

**2,000-1,000** Treat disease by balance, harmony of elements & between opposing forces of Yin & Yang • Traditional medicine develops

**551-479** K'ung Fu-tzu's (Confucius) work is based on the elements of life: water, fire, wood, metal & earth

**479-300** Revised *Nei Ching* manual of physic describes acupuncture

**c. 280** Ts'ang Kung studies medicine: writes 25 case histories

**200** Doctor Zhang Zhongjjing's massive medical book, contains all remedies & treatments known

**A.D.**

**190-265** Physician & famous surgeon, Hua Tuo pioneers abdominal surgery & use of anaesthesia. Surgical advances halt after this time, when ancient Confucian interdict on mutilation of body becomes dominant

**c. 168-196** Chang Chung-ching, Hippocrates of China, writes 16-volume classic clinical work on disease

**280** Wang Shu-ho composes 12-volume *Mei Ching* (Book of Pulse). Believes body's pulses act like musical chords

**400** Pharmacists hand down vast knowledge: belief in medical powers of precious stones & ginseng root

**1522-78** 52-volume *Great Herbal* by Li Shi-chen contains 1,900 prescriptions.

### ANCIENT EGYPT

**B.C.**

**10,000-2,000** Ancient texts provide evidence of medicine

**5,000-2,500 BC** Belief in magic: Priestly medicine

**2,900-2,750** Dentistry evidence

**2,800** Imhotep, doctor to Pharaoh Zoser • Pulse-taking

**2,500** Evidence of surgery • Knowledge of anatomy through mummification • Ptolemaic period raised ban on dissection • Doctors many and specialised • Used animal and plant extracts, more than 500 substances • Anubis: conductor of the dead

and patron god of embalmers • Surgery depicted on tombs

**1500** Physician's Tomb, Saqqara: paintings of manipulating feet and hands

**1660** Mummy of Rameses V has smallpox scars

**1600** Ebers Papyrus and Edwin Smith Papyrus – earliest known surgical text

**535** Imhotep, given full status as a god. Greeks adopt him, as Imouthes – identified with Asklepios

### ANCIENT GREECE & ROME

**B.C.**

**2000-500** Medicine is described as noble art in Homer's *Iliad*

**639-544** Thales of Miletos: 1st Greek scientist/philosopher

**580-489** Pythagoras: school at Croton • Alcmaeon of Croton

**509** Etruscans: skilled dentists

**500-428** Anaxagoras: particles theory

**500-420** Hippocrates, Father of Western Medicine. His school of medicine flourishes

**460-377** Hippocratic Oath

**c. 460** Empedocles' teaching and theory of 4 elements

**430-27** Great Plague, Athens

**400** Thucydides describes Athenian epidemic

**384-22** Aristotle founds scientific study

**370-286** Theophrastus of Eresos: *The History of Plants*

**300-200** Alexandria: Library founded by Ptolemy I

**330-260** Herophilus of Chalceon: 1st true anatomist

**234-149** Cato collects medical 'recipes'

**219** Archagathus, 1st Greek doctor in Rome, granted a public surgery & citizenship **c. 200** He founds 1st European pharmacy

**120-70** Asclepiades of Bithynia, physician, introduces humane treatment of mentally ill

**116-28** Marcus Terentius Varro recommends draining marshes

**100** Julius Caesar supposedly delivered by Caesarean section

**80** Mithridates VI experiments with poison antidotes

**48** Alexandria: Library partially destroyed by fire

**46** Julius Caesar grants citizenship to doctors in Rome

**23** Antonius Musa cures Emperor with cold water treatment • Doctors granted immunity from taxes

**A.D.**

**14-37** Celsus' *De Medicina*, earliest Latin scientific medical work describes Roman surgical/medical practice

**23-79** Pliny the Elder's *Natural History* describes many drugs

**40-90** Dioscorides describes 600 plant medicines • Vespasian frees doctors from military service

**54** Theriac, universal antidote, invented by Nero's physician, Andromarchos

**79** Vesuvius erupts • plague • 200 different medical instruments found, Pompeii

**96** Aqueducts and good water. systems: latrines, baths, drains, canals

**c. 98-117** Rufus of Ephesus writes about medicine

**c. 98-138** Soranus of Ephesus, 1st great obstetrician: his text is used for 15 centuries

**131-201** Galen, famous surgeon, writes much on anatomy, physiology and medicine – stresses humoral theory & Hippocratic doctrine

**165-69** Plague of Antoninus

**200** Medical licensing introduced

**c. 300** Guilds send texts to military forts: medical knowledge spreads

**302** Eusebius describes Syrian smallpox epidemic

**325-403** Oribasius: writes on fractures, traction and pulley systems • also medical & surgical encyclopaedia

**357-77** 1st great Christian hospital at Caesarea

**375** Plague Hospital, Edessa

**c. 397** Fabiola founds 1st hospital in Western Europe

**502-75** Aetius of Amida describes ligatures, aneurysms, diphtheria

**525-605** Alexander of Tralles: physician & author

**625-90** Paul of Aegina discusses surgical procedures

### ANCIENT INDIA

**B.C.**

**2,500-1,500** Magic important element but sorcerers become practitioners & scholars

**1,500 to 600** Charaka Samhita & Susruta Samhita, 2 basic texts of early Ayurvedic medicine. Susruta describes plastic surgery, 121 surgical instruments, 760 medical plants

**1500** Aryan invasion: Sanskrit writings about herbs, instruments, surgery

**400** Surgery extensive

**300-275** Hospitals for people & animals established

**274** Trained doctors from Taxila & Barnaras schools work with physician priests

**A.D.**

**800-1000** Brahminic medicine

**664** Moslem conquest of India: Arab medicine arrives

**1000** Ayurvedic medicine achieves modern form

### AFRICA

**BACKGROUND** The north of the continent was home to many highly civilised civilisations: the Arab world, in particular, played a large part in the advance of medicine. However, in the undiscovered interior, primitive medicine is practised for centuries. Drugs & the smearing of skin with plant substances were implemented to reduce pain during surgical procedures. Witch doctors, sometimes in a state of

trance, consult gods as to causes of disease. Treatment might involve elaborate ceremonies & there remains today a great belief in magic, charms & fetishes.

Western medicine was introduced as explorers & missionaries penetrated the 'Dark Continent'. The western coast however, was called the 'white man's grave' as so many westerners suffered from exposure to malaria – a perennial problem in Africa– & other tropical diseases.

**1284** Mausuri hospital founded in Cairo

**1348** Black Death outbreak in Egypt

**1600s** Slave trade increases spread of tropical diseases to other areas of the world

**1755** Smallpox outbreak in Cape Town: spreads inland

**1882** British control Egypt. Cultivating cash crops & new irrigation schemes mean greater exposure to water: cases of bilharzia increase

**1886** Laveran, French army surgeon working in Algeria, discovers malaria parasites

**1889** South African (Boer) War: voluntary inoculation of soldiers against typhoid

**1913** Dr Albert Schweizer, Alsatian philosopher, doctor & missionary, begins his great work in French Equatorial Africa. In due course he will build hospitals with his own hands, then equip & maintain them with money from his book royalties plus gifts from all around the world. In **1924** Schweizer returns to Africa to continue his work, creating a larger hospital & helping some 150 lepers in a leper colony (established near the hospital village that developed), using the new drugs now available

**1940s** HIV virus responsible for AIDS appears in humans

**1940** South of Cairo, 5% of population infected with *S. haematobium* in areas of basin irrigation; 60% where perennial irrigation

**1967** 1st heart transplant performed by Christiaan Barnard at Cape Town. Patient dies 18 days later

**1971** 1st combined heart & lung transplant

**1980s** HIV virus identified

**1990s** AIDS becomes pandemic. Its incidence in Africa is especially high

**1996** In Gabon 10 people die of Ebola virus after eating a chimpanzee

### AUSTRALIA

**1906** Bancroft demonstrates dengue transmitted by mosquito bites

**1912** 1st ante-natal clinic in Sydney

**1928** Flying doctor service set up in Queensland

**1976** Shannon develops bionic artificial arm

**1981** World's 1st test-tube twins born in Melbourne

**1983** 1st woman to give birth after receiving donated egg

**1984** 1st baby from a frozen embryo born in Melbourne

**1995-96** World's 1st law permitting euthanasia. 1st man dies under the voluntary euthanasia legislation

## AUSTRIA

**1365** Rudoph IV founds University of Vienna. By **1399** it has a Faculty of Medicine

**1401** 1st public dissection

**1586** University of Graz

**1672** University of Innsbruck • Theatrum anatomicum, Vienna

**1754** Van Swieten organises clinical instruction, Vienna

**1761** Auenbrugger's *Inventum novum* published

**1762** Von Plencisz's theory of *contagium animatum*

**1777-78** Frank's statistics establish importance of public health measures

**1776** Plenck's classification of skin diseases

**1783** Austria separates surgeons from barbers

**1791** University of Innsbruck restored to rank

**1810-19** Gall & Spurzheim's treatise on nervous system & skull shapes gives rise to pseudo-science of phrenology

**1839** Skoda's treatise on percussion & auscultation lays groundwork for diagnostic process

**1844** Rokitansky demonstrates tubercular nature of Pott's disease.

**1847** Semmelweis shows septicaemia causes puerperal fever • Royal Academy of Sciences, Vienna

**1862** 1st hydropathic establishment at Vienna

**1865** Mendel publishes experiments which form basis of genetic science

**1873** Billroth excises larynx

**1874** Cholera conference

**1895** Freud & Breuer publish work on 'unconscious mind'

**1879** Nitze devises electric light cystoscopy in Vienna

**1899** Gärtner's tonometer

**1900** Freud publishes *The Interpretation of Dreams*

**1901** 3 major blood cell groups described by Landsteiner • safer methods of transfusion develop

**1906** Bárány's pointing test: Nobel Prize, 1914

**1907** Von Pirquet introduces skin test for TB

**1911** Breuer proposes term 'schizophrenia'

**1940** Landsteiner & Wiener find Rh antigen in blood

## BELGIUM

**1424** 1st recorded regulations for midwives

**1426** University of Louvain

**1514-1564** Vesalius founds the 'new anatomy'

**1605** Verhoeven publishes the 1st ever newspaper

**1620** Van Helmont's *Conservation of Matter*; he founds biochemistry. In **1648** he writes *Ortus medicinae*

**1816** University of Ghent founded **1817** University of Liège founded **1834** University of Brussels

**1852 & 1876** International Congresses of Hygiene

**1897** Bordet discovers bacterial haemolysis. **1905**, with Gengou he discovers bacillus of whooping-cough.

**1906** School of Tropical Medicine, Brussels

**1920** 1st Congress of Medical History (Antwerp)

## BRITAIN

**1345** 1st apothecary shop in London • English pepperers, grocers & apothecaries unite in Guild of St Anthony

**1349** The Black Death

**1376** Board of medical examiners in London

**1460-1524** Linacre trains at Oxford & Padua: becomes kings' physician

**1485** Sweating sickness

**1500-99** Institutions for insane appear

**1505** Royal College of Surgeons of Edinburgh

**1518** Royal College of Physicians

**1540** Company of the Barber Surgeons • Henry VIII allows 4 dissections a year

**1543** English apothecaries legalised

**1547** 'Bedlam', asylum established at St Mary of Bethlehem, London

**1562** Witchcraft made capital offence **1563** Witchcraft a capital crime in Scotland

**1565** Elizabeth I permits dissection of executed criminals

**1578** William Harvey born **1616** Harvey lectures on circulation of blood

**1617** Woodall says lemon or lime juice prevent scurvy • Society of Apothecaries

**1620** Bacon's *Novum Organum*

**1624** Thomas Sydenham, 'English Hippocrates' born

**1628** Harvey publishes *De Motu Cordis* describing circulation of blood

**1643** Typhus affects armies in English Civil War

**1651** Harvey's treatise on generations of animals

**1652** Thomas Culpepper's *Herbal*

**1653** Glisson describes anatomy of liver

**1656-67** Boyle, Wren & Lower experiment with blood transfusion in animals

**1660** Willis describes puerperal fever

**1661** Scarlatina outbreak

**1662** Charles II charters Royal Society • John Graunt founds medical statistics

**1664** *Cerebri anatome* by Willis, illustrated by Wren

**1665** Great Plague of London

**1665** Hooke describes plant cells, with microscopic drawings & in **1667** shows true function of lungs

**1668-72** Dysentery epidemic

**1668** Lower shows change of colour in blood to do with uptake of substance from air

**1675** Sydenham distinguishes scarlatina from measles & discusses gout

**1689** Harris publishes work on children's diseases. **1690** Locke's *Essay on the Human Understanding* • Floyer counts the pulse by using a watch & in **1700-1710** invents special pulse watch

**1693-1694** Queen Mary II, dies of smallpox in a plague that sweeps Europe

**1703** Apothecaries authorised to prescribe drugs

**1714** Turner's treatise on skin diseases founds British dermatology

**1718** Lady Mary Wortley Montagu has son inoculated with smallpox

**1723** Yellow Fever, London

**1725** Guy's Hospital opens • 1st British school of midwifery

**1726** Hales measures blood pressure • First chair of midwifery at Edinburgh

**1730** Forceps introduced • 1st trachectomy

**1735** Witchcraft laws repealed

**1745** Barbers separated from barber surgeons

**1750** Sea Bathing Infirmary at Margate: 1st British hospital for treatment of TB

**1752** Smellie's obstetric forceps & midwifery treatise

**1743** Sir John Pringle's work on army disease

**1753** Lind's book *A Treatise on the Scurvy*

**1757** William Hunter describes arterio-venous aneurysm • Lind's treatise on naval hygiene • Brocklesby improves military conditions & sanitation

**1768** Lind's treatise on tropical medicine

**1770** William Hunter founds school of anatomy

**1771** Priestley & Scheele isolate oxygen • John Hunter's treatise on teeth & lectures on surgery

**1772** Priestley discovers nitrous oxide. Observations on different kinds of air

**1773** White urges cleanliness in midwifery to prevent puerperal fever; he pioneers asepsis

**1774** William Hunter's fine anatomical atlas published with life-size plates of human uterus • Dorset farmer, vaccinates wife & sons with cowpox • Priestley discovers ammonia

**1777** Howard's investigations of prisons & hospitals

**1779** Pott describes Pott's Disease of the Spine

**1785** John Hunter discovers collateral circulation & introduces proximal ligation • Blane's work on naval medicine

**1785** Withering's treatise on the foxglove • John Hunter's treatise on VD

**1791** Soemmerring publishes 1st volume of anatomy

**1794** John Hunter's treatises on blood, inflammation, gunshot wounds. & animal tissue transplantation

**1796** Jenner vaccinates boy with cowpox • 1798 Jenner's *Inquiry* • Willan's treatise on skin diseases

**1799** Jennerian vaccination on Continent & Asia • Hodgkin defines disease named after him

**1800** Royal College of Surgeons • Sir Humphry Davy discovers anaesthetic effect of nitrous oxide

**1803** Percival's code of medical ethics

**1811** Bell's work on spinal nerve-roots & brain anatomy

**1812** Miranda Stewart Barry qualifies as Doctor James Barrie at Edinburgh

**1817** Parkinson describes Parkinson's Disease

**1827** Richard Bright describes 'Bright's Disease'

**1830** Lister perfects achromatic microscope

**1832** British Medical Association founded • Thomas Hodgkin describes Hodgkin's Disease

**1837** Registration of deaths

**1840's** Public Health Acts mean cleaner water & mains drainage

**1841** Pharmaceutical Society of Great Britain & in 1842 its School of Pharmacy

**1847** Simpson uses chloroform

**1848** Public Health Act

**1849** Addison describes Addison's Anaemia & Addison's Disease

**1851** Great Ormond Street Hospital for Sick Children

**1853** Queen Victoria has chloroform during childbirth

**1853-56**: Crimean War. Nightingale reforms nursing

**1854** Cholera in London. John Snow proves drinking water source of infection

**1858** Medical Act: registration of doctors

**1863** Harrington invents clockwork dental drill

**1864** Parkes' Manual of Practical Hygiene

**1865** Elizabeth Garrett Anderson obtains Diploma of Society of Apothecaries

**1867** Lister operation using antiseptics • Clinical Society

**1874** London School of Medicine for Women

**1874-79** Tait: Performs 1st successful hysterectomy, & cholecsytectomy

**1875** Public Health Act

**1877** Manson shows mosquitoes transmit infective diseases

**1880** Balfour's treatise on embryology • Gower's work helps found modern neurology • London Association of Medical Women

**1883** Tait operates for ectopic pregnancy

**1886** Midwifery training given to doctors

**1888** MacEwan improves understanding of epilepsy

**1889** Infectious Diseases Notification act

**1890s** Halsted uses rubber gloves in surgery

**1890** Infectious Diseases Prevention Act

**1891** Lister Institute for Preventive Medicine

**1894** Lane introduces pinning of fractures

**1897** Ross discovers parasite responsible for malaria.

**1900** Manson's experiments prove mosquito responsible for carrying malaria • Surgical caps & masks introduced by W. Hunter

**1901** Dutton & Forde identify cause of sleeping sickness • First-ever hospital ante-natal care • King Edward VII suffers appendicitis & focuses attention of abdominal surgeons on this illness

**1902** Imperial Cancer Research Fund • Bayliss & Starling discover hormones

**1903** Bruce & Nabarro show sleeping sickness transmitted by tsetse fly • Smith perfects new operation for eye cataracts • Royal Army Medical College

**1914-18** Plastic surgery is developed by Gillies

**1915** Tetanus antitoxin for wounded soldiers

**1919** British Ministry of Health

**1920s** Marie Stopes: 1st birth-control clinic

**1924-25** London University issues external degrees for pharmacy

**1925** Insulin treatment

1928 Fleming discovers penicillin, 1st antibiotic •Vaccine against Yellow Fever

**1938** Synthetic oestrogen

**1947** All medical schools accept women

**1948** National Health Service

**1953** Crick & Watson discover structure of DNA

**1963** Human kidney transplant

**1967** Hospice care for the terminally ill

**1968** Successful heart transplant

**1969** Test tube fertilisation of human eggs

**1970** Pacemaker driven by a nuclear battery

**1972** Kidney & pancreatic tissue transplant

**1978** The world's 1st 'test-tube' baby is born

**1986** World's 1st triple heart, lungs, & liver transplant

**1997** 5-day-old baby given a new liver • Ban on the sale of beef to prevent spread of BSE 'mad cow disease' • Cloning of sheep

**1998** A 60-year old woman has a baby son

**1999** Meningitis C: vaccination campaign

## CANADA

**1639** 1st hospital

**1644** Hôtel Dieu, Montreal

**1746** Princeton College

**1821** McGill College & University founded, Montreal

**1895** Chiropractic manipulation of joints introduced by Palmer

**1906** Surgeons perform kidney operations on animals to prove human transplants possible

**1921** Insulin treatment for diabetes developed by Banting & Best

## CZECHOSLOVAKIA

**1161** Jewish physicians burned at Prague on charge of 'poisoning wells'

**1348** Clement VI charters University of Prague

**1657** Comenius publishes *Orbis pictus*

**1745** Ambulatory clinic, Prague

**1860** Czermak introduces rhinoscopy

**1867** Rokitansky performs nearly 60,000 autopsies in 50 years

**1884** Carl Koller uses cocaine in eye surgery

**1910** Jansky demonstrates 4 main blood groups: A, B, AB & O

## DENMARK

**1475** Copenhagen University

**1652** Bartholin describes lymphatic system

**1661** Stensen discovers duct of parotid gland

**1868** Meyer describes adenoid vegetations

**1893** Niels Ryberg Finsen, founder of phototherapy. demonstrates therapeutic value of actinee & ultra violet rays on skin diseases: **1903** Wins Nobel Prize

## FRANCE

**542** Nosocomia founded at Lyons & Arles

**581** Gregory of Tours describes smallpox epidemic

**590** Pandemic of St. Anthony's fire (ergotism)

**651** Hôtel-Dieu founded

**738** School of Montpellier

**962** Hospice of Great St. Bernard

**1131** Council of Rheims stops monks practising medicine for money

1180 University of Montpellier founded: **1181** it becomes a free school of medicine **1289** is chartered by Nicholas IV

**c. 1200** University of Paris

**1223-26** 2000 lazar houses

**c. 1240** Arnold of Viilanova translates Galen & Avicenna

**1257** Sorbonne founded

**1295** Lanfranch's treatise on surgery, *Cyrugia Magna*

**1300-68** Guy de Chauliac, great surgeon & leader

**1304** Henri de Mondeville teaches anatomy at Montpellier **1306** He writes his *Cyrurgia*. Develops 1st proper French surgery

**1348-50** Black Death. Guy de Chauliac helps victims. In 1363 publishes his *Chirurgia magna*

**1497-1588** Jean Fernel: introduces division of medicine into standard disciplines of physiology & pathology; 1st to describe appendicitis accurately

**1510-90** Paré, army doctor & renowned master surgeon: 1st to introduce ligatures in amputation

**1514** Pierre Brissot revives Hippocratic teaching: blood-letting near lesions

**1532** Rabelais publishes 1st Latin version of the aphorisms of Hippocrates

**1536** Paré's 1st excision of elbow-joint. In **1545** he improves amputation & gunshot wound treatment

**1551** Anatomical theatres at Paris & Montpellier

**1554** Writings by Aretaeus of Cappodocia printed

**1561** Paré founds orthopedics. *A Universal Surgery* published

**1564** Estienne & De Gorris's 2 medical dictionaries

**1567** Fernel's *Universa Medicinia* – includes a section on therapeutics

**1575** Paré introduces massage & artificial eyes

**1578** De Baillou describes whooping cough

**1596** Descartes born. In **1637** he shows visual accommodation depends on change in form of lens. In **1644** he describes reflex action & publishes treatise on dioptrics. In **1662** 1st treatise on physiology

**1609** Louise Bourgeois publishes her observations on midwifery

**1656** Lazar houses abolished

**1667** Jean Baptiste Denis of Paris transfuses blood from lamb to man

**1674** More's tourniquet for checking haemorrhage

**1678-1761** Fauchard, known as 'father of dentistry'. Writes *The Surgeon Dentist, A Treatise on Teeth*, describing oral anatomy & pathology, plus dental techniques

**1679** De Blegny publishes 1st medical periodical *Nouvelles découvertes*

**1683** Duverney's 1st treatise on otology

**1705** Brisseau & Maitre Jan show cataract is a clouded lens

**1713** Anel catheterises tear ducts. **1714** He invents fine point syringe

**1715** Petit differentiates between compression and concussion of brain

**1720-21** Plague in Marseilles • Palfyn's obstetric forceps

**1724** De Moivre publishes memoir *Annuities upon lives* • Guyot of Versailles attempts catheterisation of Eustachian tubes

**1728** Fauchard's *Le chirurgien dentiste*

**1730** Réamur introduces 80 degree thermometer

**1731** Hoffmann describes chlorosis • 1st Academy of Surgeons

**1736** Petit 1st to open mastoid, & perform a cholecystectomy

**1739** Morand makes 1st excision of hip-joint

**1741** André calls study of bones orthopaedics

**1745** Deparcieux's idea of 'mean expectation of life'

**1749** Buffon's *Natural History* • Senac's treatise on the heart

**1752** Réaumur's experiments on digestion in birds

**1753** Daviel's modern method of cataract extraction

**1764** Louis claims to introduce digital compression for haemorrhage

**1766** Cavendish discovers hydrogen • Desault's bandage for fractures

**1770** Abbé de l'Épée invents sign language for deaf-mutes

**1771-1802** Bichat shows how individual tissue can be diseased. *Anatomie générale, apliquée à la physiologie et à médicine* is one of medicine's most important books

**1777** Lavoisier describes exchange of gases in respiration

**1779** Mesmer's memoir on animal magnetism

**1783** Marschal excises prolapsed cancerous uterus

**1786** Moreau excises elbow-joint

**1793** Larrey introduces *ambulances volantes*

**1794** Lavoisier guillotined

**1800s** Dupuytren: important in anatomy & pathology; performs daring surgery; devises new instruments

**1800-01** Seen as founding modern histology & tissue pathology, Bichat's *Traité des membranes* & *Anatomie générale*. He revolutionises descriptive anatomy • Cuvier's *Comparative Anatomy* • Pinel's psychiatric treatise. He reforms treatment of insane

**1812** Larrey 1st uses local anaesthesia by freezing limbs before amputation. His care for patients will form basis of Red Cross

**1815-19** Laënnec invents stethoscope

**1818** Pelletier & Caventou isolate strychnine & quinine

**1820** Coindet uses iodine in goiter

**1821** Itard's treatise on otology

**1822-40** Magendie pioneers physiology & pharmacology, studies spinal canal & nervous system; demonstrates Bell's law of the spinal nerve roots: analyses drug action

**1823** Chevreul investigates animal fats

**1824** Flouren works on cerebral physiology

**1825** Bouillaud describes & localises aphasia

**1825-93** Charcot researches epilepsy & other neurological diseases. Works at Salpêtrière hospital in Paris

**1826** Laënnec gives classical description of bronchitis & other thoracic diseases

**1827** Seglas invents endoscope

**1829** Braille introduces printing for the blind

**1831** Soubeiran discovers chloroform

**1834** Dumas obtains & names pure chloroform

**1835** Louis founds medical statistics • Cruveilhier describes multiple sclerosis

**1840s** A founder of endocrinology, Brown-Séquard demonstrates function of suprenal gland: 1st scientist to work out physiology of spinal card & to discover hormones

**1846-49** Bernard describes digestive function of pancreas, & glycogenic function of liver in sugar metabolism; produces diabetes by puncturing fourth ventricle • Magendie pioneers physiology & pharmacology

**1851-54** Bernard describes vasomotor function of sympathetic nervous system: discovers function of vaso-dilator nerves

**1858** Marey: 1st to show vagus tone increases with increase of blood pressure so can assess absolute pressure of blood in a human artery • Bernard discovers vaso-constrictor & extended vaso-dilator nerves

**1860** Ménière describes aural vertigo, severe giddiness (Ménière's Disease)

**1861** Pasteur discovers anaerobic bacteria • Broca says speech control located in brain's left frontal lobe

**1863** Pasteur discovers bacteria destroyed by heat; invents pasteurisation; investigates silkworm disease

**1865** Villemin demonstrates TB due to specific agent he calls a 'germ'

**1867** Bernard establishes principle of homeostasis

**1869-72** Universities accept woman medical students

**1874** *Loi Roussel* enacted for protection of infants

**1878** International Congress of Hygiene

**1880-81** Pasteur isolates streptococcus, staphylococcus & pneumococcus • Laveran discovers malarial fever parasite

**1883-6** Pasteur vaccinates against anthrax; makes 1st effective vaccine against rabies, *Méthode pour prévenir la rage*

**1886** Neurologist, Pierre Marie describes gigantism due to pituitary gland disease

**1887** D'Arsonval introduces high frequency currents

**1888** Institut Pasteur founded • Roux & Yersin investigate diphtheria toxins

**1894** Kitasato & Yersin discover plague bacillus

**1896** Becquerel discovers radioactivity in uranium • Widal & Sicard introduce agglutination test for typhoid fever

**1898** Pierre & Marie Curie discover radium

**1900** Widal & Ravaut introduce cytodiagnosis

**1902** Carre introduces vascular anastomosis & transplantation of tissues

**1903** Metchnikoff inoculates higher apes with syphilis

**1905** Psychologist, Binet, develops way of testing brain's ability to reason

**1907** Laveran awarded Nobel prize • Calmette devises conjunctival test for TB • In Paris, doctors announc discovery of a serum to cure dysentery

**1910** Victor Henri & others introduce ultraviolet sterilisation of water • Gattefossé studies therapeutic actions of plant oils • Marie Curie's treatise on radiography

**1911** Carrel investigates extravital culture & rejuvenation of tissues

**1912** Dastre pioneers cornea graft to restore eyesight • Odin claims isolation & cultivation of cancer microbe

**1913** De Sandfort devises ambrine (paraffin-resin solution) treatment for burns

**1914-18** Carrel & Dakin improve treatment of infected wounds

**1921** Development of TB vaccine from living non-virulent bovine bacilli by Calmette & Guérin; **1924** introduced as BCG preventive vaccination

**1926** Pasteur Institute announces discovery of antitetanus serum

**1950** Küss & colleagues transplant kidneys from deceased to living patients

**1998** 1st arm transplant operation

## GERMANY

**1163** Abbess, Hildegard von Bingen, writes on holistic healing & natural history

**1193-1280** Albertus Magnus, dominant in science learning

**1316** City surgeon at Lübeck earns 16 marks per annum

**1440** Printing press: Gutenberg uses movable type for 1st time

**1457** Tutenberg Purgation-Calendar 1st medical publication

**1469-78** Da Grado's *Practica* & Mondino's *Anathomia*

**1484** Schhöffer's herbal *Latin Herbarius* • 1485 German Herbarius

**1493** Smallpox outbreak

**1513** Rösslin's *Roszgarten* - earliest printed text book for midwives

**1517** Fugitive anatomical plates published by Schott of Mainz • Gersdorff's *Field-Book of Wound-Surgery*

**1518** Nuremberg ordinance regulating sale of food

**1522** Doctor Wertt of Hamburg burned at stake for impersonating a midwife

**1530** Brunfels' atlas of plants, *Herbarium vivae eicones*

**1542** Fuchs herbal classifying medical plants

**1546** Cordus's pharmacopoeia • Bock's *Kräuterbuch*

**1560-1634** Father of German Surgery, Wilhelm Fabry, amputates with red-hot knife to reduce haemorrhage & through healthy tissue above gangrenous parts (rather than into gangrene)

**1583** Bartisch's *Augendienst* 1st book on eye surgery

**1604** Kepler shows inversion of optic image on retina

**1619** Scheiner's *Oculus*

**1640** Rolfink revives dissecting ('rolfinken')

**1642** Wirsung discovers pancreatic duct named after him

**1653-55** Scultetus's *Armamentarium chirurgicum* shows graphic representation of breast amputation

**1660** Schneider shows nasal secretion not from pituitary body

**1680** Plague hospital in Magdeburg

**1690** Siegemundin's treatise on midwifery

**1698** Stahl's treatise on diseases of the portal system: In **1702** he states phlogiston theory

**1713** Theatrum anatomicum, Berlin

**1714** Fahrenheit makes 212 degree mercury thermometer

**1716** Surgeon General appointed in German Army at 900 marks per annum

**1719** Heister's work on surgery – founder of German scientific surgery

**1721** General Holtzendorff creates 'Collegium medico-chirurgicum' at Berlin

**1738** Lieberkühn invents reflector microscope

**1740** Hoffman describes rubella

**1745** Kratzenstein uses electrotherapy

**1751** Königliche Gesellschaft der Wissenschaften at Göttingen founded by Haller

**1754** 1st woman with medical doctorate, at Halle

**1756** Frederick the Great's dentist, Pfaff, describes making plaster models from wax impressions

**1755-1843** Samuel Hahnemann; he becomes founder of homeopathy

**1757** Halle's *Elementa physiologiae corporis humani et causis morborum*

**1762** Roederer & Wagler describe typhoid fever

**1768** Wolff's classic on chick's intestine embryology

**1778** Von Siebold performs symphysiotomy

**1781** Kant's *Critique of Pure Reason*

**1791** Soemmering publishes 1st volume of his anatomy

**1795** Frank's 7 volumes *De curandis hominum morbis epitome*

**1805-06** Sertürner isolates morphine

**1807** Compulsory vaccination introduced in Bavaria & Hesse

**1828** Forerunner of organic chemistry, Wöhler synthesises urea

**1830** Kopp describes thymus-death

**1831-02** Von Liebig discovers chloroform, analyses acetone & discovers chloral

**1833** Müller's physiology treatise

**1836** Schwann discovers pepsin in stomach. In **1841** he shows bile essential for digestion. Great work on nerves & muscles

**1837** Henle describes epithelial tissues of skin & intestine. Contributes greatly to microscopic anatomy • Schönlein publishes *Peliosis Rheumatica*, describing skin condition of purpura known by his name • Schwann discovers yeast cell & founds a germ theory

**1838** Schleiden describes plant cells • Johannes Müller's treatise on tumours

**1839** Schwann publishes treatise on cell theory

**1840s** Wunderlich uses a clinical thermometer

**1841** Henle's *Allgemeine Anatomie* contains many of his discoveries

**1842** Wöhler describes synthesis of hippuric from benzoic acid. • Dieffenbach's treatise on strabismus

**1843** Ludwig investigates urinary secretion mechanism

**1845-58** Creator of modern pathology, Virchow discovers much about human cell, & with Bennett, describes leukemia. He shows embolism is cause of pyaemia • Langenbeck detects actinomyces

**1846** Weber brothers discover inhibitory effect of vagus nerve

**1848-51** Helmholtz locates source of animal heat in muscles; measures velocity of nerve current; invents ophthalmoscope for examination of eye interior • Du Bois-Reymond's treatise on animal electricity

**1854** Virchow describes neuroglia

**1857** Graefe introduces operation for strabismus

**1854** Virchow's *Die Cellular Pathologie*: founds cellular pathology • Niemann isolates cocaine

**1859** Kirchhoff & Bunsen develop recording spectroscope • Kolbe synthesises salicylic acid

**1861** Max Schultze defines protoplasm & cell

**1862** F. Hoppe Seyler discovers haemoglobin

**1863** Preparation of barbituric acid by Van Baeyer • Helmholtz's *Tonempfindungen* • Voit & Pettenkofer's investigations of metabolism in respiration

**1866** Voit establishes 1st hygienic laboratory, Munich

**1867** Helmholtz's treatise on physiological optics

**1868** Haeckel's *Natürliche Schöpfungsgeschichte* • Wunderlich's work on temperature in disease founds clinical thermometer

**1869** Esmarch introduces india rubber bandage to provide bloodless field for limb surgery • Virchow urges medical inspection of schools

**1869-72** Universities accept women medical students

**1870** Simon reports successful planned removal of kidney

**1871** Weigert stains bacteria with carmine

**1872** Abbe introduces optical instruments & oil immersion lenses • Billroth excises larynx • Revaccination compulsory • Obermeier discovers spirillum of relapsing fever

**1874** Ehrlich introduces dried blood smears & improves stain methods

**1875** Lösch discovers *Entamolba histolytica*, infective agent of amoebic dysentery • Meat inspection compulsory • Landois discovers haemolysis

**1876** Imperial Board of Health founded, Berlin • Koch grows anthrax bacilli on artificial medium & isolates salicylic acid

**1877** Cohnheim: successful inoculation of TB in rabbit's eye • Nitze introduces cystoscopy

**1878** Von Volkmann successfully removes a rectum cancer • Freund excises cancerous uterus • Koch discovers causes of traumatic infections

**1879** Neisser discovers gonococcus • German food law passed

**1881-82** Billroth resects pylorus • Koch introduces plate cultures & discovers tubercle bacillus •Flemming studies cell division

**1883-84** Klebs discovers diphtheria bacillus •Koch discovers cholera bacillus

**1885** Weismann's memoir on continuity of germ plasm • Weigert begins hematoxylin staining of nerve-fibres

**1886** Von Bergmann begins steam sterilisation in surgery

**1887** Flick invents glass contact lenses

**1889-90** Von Behring discovers anti-toxins • Buchner discovers alexins • Von Mering & Minkowski produce experimental pancreatic diabetes •Von Behring & Kitasato discover diphtheria & tetanus antitoxins & provide basis for serotherapy • Von Behring treats diphtheria with antitoxin •Koch introduces tuberculin • Weigert stains neurolglia with methyl violet

**1891** Institute for Infectious Diseases, Berlin, under Koch • Waldeyer founds neuron theory • Quinke uses lumbar puncture

**1892** Cholera epidemic in Hamburg • Kossel & Neumann discover pentose

**1893** Aspirin marketed, to treat rheumatism • International Cholera Conference, Dresden

**1895** Röntgen discovers x-rays; takes 1st x-ray of his wife's hand • His reforms anatomical nomenclature

**1897** Fischer synthesises caffeine, theobromine, xanthin, guanin & adenin

**1898** Löffler & Frosch investigate filtrable viruses • Fischer isolates purin nucleus of uric acid compounds •Heroin & aspirin used in medicine

**1899** Einhorn synthesis of procaine (novocaine) • Ehrlich's Institute for serology & serum testing becomes Royal Institute for experimental therapy at Frankfurt. Ehrlich's work there founds chemotherapy

**1900** Wertheim introduces radical operation for uterine cancer

**1901** Koch states that bubonic plague may have been due to solely to rats • Röntgen wins Nobel Prize

**1902** Earbituric acid formula patented

**1903** Fischer & Von Mering introduce veronal • Bier introduces artificial hyperemia in surgery

**1904** Sauerbruch designs negative pressure chamber for surgery of chest

**1905** Schaudinn discovers spirochaete of syphilis • Koch studies African fever

**1907** Wassermann introduces sero diagnostic test for syphilis

**1909** Ehrlich introduces Salvarsan. In **1911** he tests it in the treatment of syphilis – seen as the birth of chemotherapy

**1912** Sudhoff opposes theory of American origin of syphilis, believing it existed in Europe pre-Columbus

**1917** Von Economo describes experimental transmission of encephalitis lethargica

**1928** Ascheim & Zondek introduce 1st usable pregnancy test

1932 Anti-malarial drug, atebrin, synthesised by Mietzsch, Mauss & Kikuth • Evipan, a barbiturate anaesthetic, introduced by Weese & Scharpff • 1st electron-microscope

**1935** Domagh finds that pronotosil protects mice against fatal doses of striptococcol

**1979** 1st human liver transplant

## IRELAND

**675** Monastic records of smallpox

**1593** University of Dublin (Trinity College) founded

**1770** Rutty describes relapsing fever

**1784** Royal College of Surgeons in Ireland

**1785** Chair of anatomy in University of Dublin

**1827** Adams describes heart-block

**1832** Corrigan describes aortic insufficiency

**1835** Graves urges use of healthy nutritious foods. Gives classic account of exuphthalmic goitre now known as Graves Disease

**1837** Colles states law of maternal immunity in syphilis

**1845** Rynd invents instrument to give hypodermic infusions • Potato Famine – thousands emigrate

## ITALY

**848-56** Hospital from which School of Salerno will develop by tenth century, with women professors. The best known was Trotula, a gynaecologist, who published a book on midwifery

**1020-87** Constantinus the African. Medieval medical scholar translates Greek & Arabic works into Latin

**1025** University of Parma

**1080-1200** School of Salerno a centre of knowledge. 5-year courses of study. Anatomical dissection on animals

**1140** Roger II of Sicily restricts medical practice to licentiates

**1150-58** Medical school & University of Bologna

**1170** Roger of Palermo completes *Cyrurgia Rogerii*

**1180** Roger of Parma's *Practica chirurgiae*

**1201-77** Saliceto: surgeon, writes many books

**1221** Frederick II decrees no-one to practise medicine unless approved by masters of Salerno. In **1224** he issues law regulating study of medicine; founds Naples & Messina Universities **1231** authorises a quinquennial dissection at Salerno **1240-41** makes regulations – to separate pharmacy from medicine; institute government supervision of pharmacy; oblige pharmacists to take an oath to prepare drugs reliably: to encourage dissection

**1250** Roland of Parma, edits Roger of Salerno's work

**1260** De Mondeville, surgeon to Philip the Fair, advises cleanliness & describes surgical procedures

**1266** Borgognoni or Theodeoric teaches new treatment of wounds

**1267** Council of Venice forbids Jews to practice medicine among Christians

**1270** Spectacles introduced by Venetian glassmakers

**1275** Saliceto completes treatise on regional surgical anatomy; advocates knife rather than usual cautery

**1295** Lanfranchi's treatise on surgery, *Cyrugia Magna*

**1302** 1st judicial post-mortem, at Bologna

**1315** Anatomical dissection by De Luzzi at Bologna

**1316** Mondino writes 1st 'modern' text book on anatomy *Anathomia*

**1317** Bull against alchemy & other magical practices

**1345** *Anatomica* by Guido de Vigrevano tries to improve status of surgeons

**1400s** Boards of Health at Venice & Milan

**1450** Krebs suggests time pulse & weighing of blood & urine

**1472** Bagellardo's treatise on paediatrics

**1474-78** Saliceto's *Cyrurgia* (work on surgery & 1st edition of work of Celsus printed: 1st medical author printed in moveable type

**1497** Aldine edition of Theophrastus printed

**1498** Florentine *Ricettario* (1st official pharmacopoeia)

**1500** Da Carpi treats syphilis with mercury

**1507** Benivieni's collection of post-mortem sections printed

**1510** Leonardo da Vinci's fine drawings of human body

**1521-23** Da Carpi publishes anatomical treatises

**1523-62** Fallopius teaches at Padua, writes on anatomy, studies reproductive system & inner ear. Fallopian tubes are named after him

**1526** 1st (Aldine) Greek translation of Hippocrates

**1530** Fracastorius' poem on syphilis published

**1535** Mariano Santo di Barletta: 1st account of median lithotomy

**1537** Dryander's *Anatomia*

**1537-1619** Fabricius ab Aquapedente discovers much about valves in veins

**1538** Vesalius publishes his *Tabulae anatomicae sex*

**1540** Mattioli: internal use of mercury for syphilis

**1543** Vesalius founds modern anatomy: *De Humani Corporis Fabrica*

**1546** Fracastoro publishes work on contagious illnesses

**1549** Anatomy theatre, Padua

**1558** Cornaro's treatise on personal hygiene

**1559** Comuno describes pulmonary circulation

**1561** Fallopius (Fallopio) *Observationes anatonmicae*, greatly extends knowledge of anatomy, especially female reproductive system, inner ear, cerebral arteries, nerves, eye muscles, tissues

**1564** Galileo born. Develops careful measurement in medicine, microscope & telescope • Eustachius discovers abducens nerve thoracic duct & suprarenal glands

**1567** Paracelsus' account of miners' phthisis

**1572** Mercuriale's systematic treatise on skin diseases

**1576** Paracelsus's tract on mineral waters

**1580** Alpino introduces moxabustion from Orient

**1586** Della Porta's *De humana physiognomia* pioneers physiogynomy

**1594** 1st permanent operating theatre at Padua

**1595** Quercetanus uses purgative, calomel • Mercurio's *La Comare o Raccoglitrice* (The Midwife)

**1597** Tagliacozzi's treatise on plastic surgery

**1603** Fabricus ab Aquapendente's *De Venarium Ostiolis* suggests to Harvey the circulation of the blood

**1609** Clinical thermometer invented by Sanctorius

**1610** Galileo's microscope

**1622** Aselli discovers lacteal vessels

**1626** Sanctorius Santonio records use of clinical thermometer & pulse clock

**1629** Severino makes 1st resection of wrist

**1633-1717** Ramazzini: Writes 1st full-scale treatise on occupational health

**1640** Severino creates local anaesthesia with snow & ice

**1648** Kircher describes ear trumpet • Redi disproves spontaneous generation theory

**1654-1720** Maria discusses idea that malaria might be caused by mosquito bites

**1658** Kircher attributes plague to *contagium animatum*

**1659-61** Malpighi outlines lymphadenoma; discovers capilliary anastomosis; describes histology of lungs

**1662** Bellini discovers kidneys' excretory ducts

**1666** Malpighi's treatise on viscera. **1670** He discovers Malpighian bodies in spleen & kidneys. **1673** He describes chick development. **1675** Publishes *Anatome plantarum*

**1680-81** Borelli studies mechanics & 'physical laws' of the body; publishes *De motu animalium*

**1682-1771** Examination of dead body developed by pathologist Morgagni

**1700** Ramazzini's treatise on occupational diseases

**1704** Valsalva describes Valsalva's manoeuvre

**1710** Santorini's muscle in larynx discovered

**1719** Morgagni describes syphilis of cerebral arteries

**1761** Morgagni's *De sedibus*

**1770** Cotugno demonstrates albumen in urine

**1772** Scarpa discovers ear labyrinth

**1784** Cotugno discovers cerebro-spinal fluid

**1787** Mascagni publishes atlas of lymphatics

**1794** Scarpa's *Tabulae nevrologicae* shows his work on heart nerves. In **1804** he describes arteriosclerosis

**1827** Amici & Cuthbert invent reflecting microscope

**1876** Lombroso inaugurates doctrine of 'criminal type"

**1916** Vanghetti introduces cineplasty

## JAPAN

**1868** University of Tokyo

**1890** Kitasato & Von Behring discover diphtheria & tetanus antitoxins

**1894** Kitasato & Yersin discover plague bacillus

**1897** Shiga discovers dysentery bacillus

**1909** Noguchi improves the Wassermann reaction: **1911** introduces luetin reaction: **1913** demonstrates Spirochaete pallida in brains of syphilitic patients suffering from paresis: **1920** discovers leptospira in Yellow Fever: **1928** dies of Yellow Fever in Ghana

**1914-1915** Inada & others describe cause, method of infection & treatment of spirochaetal jaundice

**1916** Futaki & others discover a spirillum in cases of ratbite fever

**1920** Naito's artificial blood

## NETHERLANDS

**1590** Invention of compound microscope by Hans & Zacharia Janssen

**1621** Drebbel improves microscope

**1638** Drebbel improves thermometer

**1642-45** Cholera 1st studied by Bonitus who also describes beriberi in his book *De medicina Indorum*

**1646** Diemerbroek publishes monograph on plague

**1658** Swammerdam describes red blood-corpuscles

**1662** De Graaf shows that ova arise in the ovary

**1663** Sylvius describes digestion as a fermentation

**1664** Swammerdam discovers valves of lymphatics • De Graaf examines pancreatic juice & its importance in digestion of food In **1667** he describes docimiasia of fetal lungs

**1670** Swammerdam discovers muscle-tonus

**1672** De Graaf describes Graafian follicles in ovary

**1673** Leeuwenhoek makes microscopes & describes red blood cells. In **1683** he describes bacteria. Discoveries: **1674** sperm; **1675** protozoa; **1679** striped muscle; **1680** yeast plant; **1689** rods in retina & finer anatomy of cornea; **1703** parthenogenesis of plant lice

**1732** Boerhaave's *Elementa chemiae*

**1738** Lieberkühn invents reflector microscope

**1758** De Haën uses thermometer in clinical work

**1860** Donders introduces cylindrical & prismatic spectacles for astigmatism. In **1862** he publishes studies on astigmatism & presbyopia

**1869-72** Universities accept women medical students

**1901** De Vries's mutation theory

**1903** Einthoven invents string galvanometer, 1st practical electrocardiograph (ECG) • Rocci invents sphygmomanometer for measuring blood pressure

**1910** Worldwide organisation Féderation Internationale Pharmaceutique begins

**1924** Einthoven wins Nobel Prize

**1930** Debye uses x-rays to investigate molecule structure • 1st kidney dialysis machine developed by Kolff in secret for Dutch resistance

## RUSSIA

**1755** University of Moscow

**1798** Imperial Medico-Military Academy, St Petersburg

**1819** University of St Petersburg

**1852** Pirogoff uses frozen sections in his *Anatome topigraphica*

**1867** Pavlov, famous for his dogs, helps understanding of conditioned reflexes

**1892** Ivanovsky describes mosaic tobacco disease & discovers viruses

**1937** Artificial heart by Demikhov

**1970** Balloon surgery

## SOUTH AMERICA

In earliest times, Pre Columbian medicine is a mix of religious & magical practice. Tropical forests remain a source of many drugs

**1508** Guaiac from West Indies & Tropical America used as wood or resin for syphilis, dropsy & gout

**1524** Cortes erects 1st hospital in city of Mexico

**1530s** Sarsaparilla – dried roots of several tropical American plants – used as an emetic, to treat psoriasis, & as flavouring

**1609** Jalap, a purgative from the fibrous roots of a climbing plant, brought to Europe from Mexico

**1721** Universidad central de Venezuela, Caracas

**1743** University of Santiago founded in Chile

**1808** Medical Faculty at Rio de Janeiro, Brazil

**1901** Instituto Oswaldo Cruz, Rio de Janeiro, Brazil

## SPAIN & PORTUGAL

**580** Hospital at Merida founded by Bishop Masona

**936** Albucasis, Muslim surgeon, writes 1st illustrated book on surgery & introduces using red hot iron to cauterise wounds

**1094-1162** Ibn Zuhr, Arab physician born in Seville. Writes treatise on clinical medicine

**1309** University of Coimbra chartered by King Diniz of Portugal (reconstituted, 1772). An important school of medicine

**1391** University of Lerida permitted to dissect a body every 3 years • 1st dissection recorded in Spain

**1400s** Gold leaf used as a dental filling material

**1409** Insane asylum at Seville; & **1425** Insane asylum, Saragossa

**1450** University of Barcelona
**1501** University of Valencia
**1504** University of Santiago
**1505** University of Seville
**1508** University of Madrid
**1531** University of Granada

**1537** Dryander's *Anatomia*

**1548** Charles V declares surgery honourable

**1553** Servede, 1st to suggest transit of blood through lungs, burnt at stake in Geneva because of his revolutionary ideas

**1571** Bravo describes Spanish typhus

**1583-1600** Diphtheria (garotillo) epidemic

**1590** D'Acosta describes mountain sickness

**1611** Real & Vilius describe diphtheria (garotillo) epidemic

**1638** Acuna, Portuguese monk, uses oil of capaiva

**1640** Malaria arrives • Del Vigo introduces cinchona, a substitute from Peruvian bark associated with quinine & a cure for fevers

**1935** 1st pre-frontal leucotomy by Moniz to treat some psychoses

## SWEDEN

**1735** Linnaeus's *Systema naturae*

**1742** Celsius invents 100 degree thermometer •Linnaeus describes aphasia & then in **1763** publishes his classification of disease, *Genera morborum*

**1764** Von Rosenstein of Uppsala's book on children's diseases & treatment begins modern paediatrics

**1774** Scheele discovers chlorine •**1776** with Bergmann, he discovers uric acid in bladder stones

**1808** Swedish Medical Society

**1869-72** Universities accept female medical students

**1880** Sandström describes parathyroid gland

**1911** Gullstrand wins Nobel prize for optical researches

**1958** Ake Senning implants 1st internal heart pacemaker

**1956** Fijoe & Levan state 46 normal human chromosomes exist. Leads to discovery of Down's Syndrome

## SWITZERLAND

**1460** University of Basel founded by citizens of city

**1493-1551** Paracelsus: questions classics & defies tradition; advocates chemical therapies, called the 'father of pharmacology'. In **1527** he publishes his revolutionary ideas, promises to free medicine from its worst errors & burns books by Galen & Avicenna

**1537** Vesalius graduates, Basel

**1554** Rueff's *De Conceptu*, becomes popular handbook for midwives

**1570** Platter, one of 1st to distinguish between various mental disorders, urges psychic treatment of insane

**1588** Anatomy theatre, Basel

**1602** Platter publishes 1st attempt at classification of diseases. He dissects more than 300 bodies

**1623** Medical Faculty added to University of Altdorf

**1658** Wepfer demonstrates lesion of brain in apoplexy

**1677** Peyer describes lymphoid follicles in small intestine, Peyer's patches

**1682** Brunner describes duodenal glands, found **1679** by father-in-law, Wepfer

**1708-77** Von Haller, writer, botanist, physiologist, who studies nervous system. In **1736** he points out function of bile in digestion of fats

**1739** Royal Swedish Academy of Medicine

**1744** Trembley describes regeneration of tissues in hydrozoa

**1747** Haller's *Primae lineae physiologiae*, 1st textbook on physiology

**1749** Meyer orders phthisical patients to mountain areas

**1752** Haller publishes memoir of specific irritability of tissues. **1757** publishes his *Elementa physiologiae corporis humani et causis morborum*

**1805** Vieusseux describes cerebro-spinal meningitis

**1832** University of Zurich **1834** University of Bern

**1846** Kölliker describes smooth muscle. In **1852** his *Handbuch der Gwewbelenhre* is 1st systematic treatise on histology

**1865** Universities accept women medical students

**1948** World Health Organisation forms, Geneva

**1972** Borel discovers cyclosporin-A from a mushroom suppresses immune system & helps transplants to take

### USA AND CANADA

**1636** Harvard College founded by act of General Court of Massachusetts. • Assembly of Virginia passes act regulating surgeons' fees

**1638** Assembly of Maryland act regulates surgeons' fees

**1639** 1st hospital in Canada • Virginia Assembly's law regulates medical practice

**1646** Syphilis in Boston

**1647** Yellow Fever in Barbados spreads through American ports • Firmin lectures on anatomy in Massachusetts

**1649** Act regulates medical practice in Massachusetts

**1659** Diphtheria at Roxbury, Massachusetts

**1663** 1st hospital in American colonies (Long Island, N.Y.)

**1666** Coroners appointed for each county of Maryland

**1668** Yellow Fever, New York

**1677** Smallpox in Boston

Printing presses: **1674** Boston; **1681** Williamsburg, Virginia; **1685** Philadelphia; **1693** New York

**1685** Bidloo's *Anatomia* • Vieussens' *Nevrographia* on brain, spinal cord & nerves. Best illustrated 17th-century work on subject

**1691** Autopsy of Governor Slaughter in New York • Yellow fever in Boston

**1692** Salem Witchcraft Trials

**1699** Infectious diseases act in Massachusetts

**1703-1850** Devastating epidemics of Yellow Fever in tropical/subtropical zones

**1716** New York City issues ordinance for midwives

**1717** Hospital for infectious diseases, Boston

**1721** Boylston inoculates for smallpox in Boston

**1730-31** Cadwalader teaches anatomy in Philadelphia

**1735** Scarlatina appears

**1760** W. Shippen, Jr., lectures on anatomy in Philadelphia • Act regulates medical practice in New York

**1762** 1st medical library in USA (Pennsylvania Hospital) • Shippen's private maternity hospital, Philadelphia

**1765** John Morgan founds 1st medical school in USA at College of Pennsylvania

**1768** Medical School Kings College, New York

**1770** 1st medical degree in USA conferred by King's College on Robert Tucker • Pennsylvania quarantine act

**1772** New Jersey act regulates medical practice

**1773** 1st insane asylum in USA, Williamsburg, Virginia

**1774** Chovet teaches anatomy in Philadelphia

**1777** William Shippen: Director General of American Army Medical Department

**1778** Brown publishes 1st USA pharmacopoeia *Pharmacopoeia simpliciorum et efficaciorum* • Yellow Fever, Memphis

**1780** Benjamin Franklin invents bifocal lenses • Dengue fever at Philadelphia

**1782** Medical Department of Harvard University founded

**1787** College of Physicians of Philadelphia

**1791-99** Baynham, operates for extra-uterine pregnancy

**1796** Yellow Fever in Boston • Wright Post successfully ligates femoral artery

**1797** Medical Repository (New York) published

**1797-99** Yellow Fever in Philadelphia

**1798** Medical & Chirurgical Faculty of Maryland founded

**1800** Waterhouse introduces Jennerian vaccination in New England

**1809** Famous surgeon, McDowell of Kentucky performs ovariotomy

**1810** Yale Medical School

**1812** *Medical inquiries & observations upon the diseases of the*

*mind* by Rush, 1st American book on psychiatry • Bellevue Hospital, New York

**1817** Plantson invents dental plate

**1820** 1st American Pharmacopoeia published

**1821** Philadelphia College of Pharmacy, 1st in USA

**1825** Fever hospital, New York City

**1828-1917** Dr Andrew Taylor Still; will found osteopathy

**1831** Guthrie discovers chloroform

**1831-1915** Black reforms dentistry – devises foot engine so dentists can keep both hands free when powering drill. Notes densely matted coating on teeth & suggests dental caries & periodontal disease infections brought about by bacteria. Scientific evidence confirms this – but not until 1960s!

**1832** Cholera: 3 major outbreaks during century • Boston Lying-in Hospital

**1833** Beaumont publishes experiments on digestion

**1839-40** Baltimore College of Dental Surgery is 1st dental school in world

**1842** Long operates with ether anaesthesia

**1843** Holmes writes *Contagiousness of puerperal fever* – a medical classic

**1846** Morton uses ether to put patient to sleep during dental operation • J. Marion Sims invents a vaginal speculum

**1847** 1st school for mentally retarded, in Massachusetts

**1847** American Medical Association • New York Academy of Medicine

**1849** 1st English woman to graduate as a doctor: Elizabeth Blackwell, at the Geneva Medical School, New York • J. M. Sims operates for vesico-vaginal fistula

**1850** Detmold opens abscess of brain

**1852** American Pharmaceutical Association

**1853** Sims's treatise on vesicovaginal fistula In **1855** founds Hospital for Women's Diseases, New York

**1861** Wollcott (Milwaukee) 1st excises renal tumour

**1861-65** American Civil War. Many outbreaks of communicable disease • Beaumont treats war patient's close shotgun blast: he survives with permanent exterior opening to stomach

**1865** Chicago Hospital for Women

**1866** Sims's *Clinical Notes on Uterine Surgery*

**1875** Silas Weir Mitchell's rest cure for nervous diseases • Boston Medical Library

**1876** Johns Hopkins University: many forward-thinking investigative & innovative policies

**1880** American Surgical Association founded

**1884** Koller uses cocaine in eye surgery

**1886** Fitz describes pathology of appendicitis

**1889** Johns Hopkins Hospital (Baltimore) opens

**1890** Halsted introduces rubber gloves for surgery at Johns Hopkins

**1892** Welsh & Nuttall discover gas gangrene bacillus • Halsted ligates subclavian artery in 1st portion

**1895** Chiropractic manipulation of joints introduced by Palmer

**1897** Cannon's solution of radio-opaque bismuth acts as diagnostic meal to outline stomach • Murphy: 1st to successfully repair gunshot wound of a major artery

**1897-98** Cannon discovers barium suspensions show alimentary canal on x-ray plate

**1898** Pathologist T. Smith differentiates between bovine & human tubercle bacilli

**1899** Reed, Carroll, Simoni & Lazear establish transmission of Yellow Fever by mosquito

**1899** Loeb produces chemical activation of sea urchin egg

**1901** Rockefeller Institute for Medical Research, New York

**1902** North & South America establish International Sanitary Bureau

**1903** Henry Phipps Institute for Tuberculosis, Baltimore • Porcelain fillings

**1904** Atwater invents respiration calorimeter

**1906** Nutrition Laboratory, Boston • 'Typhoid Mary', famous typhoid carrier, discovered • Food & Drugs Act

**1907** Immigrants health checks to ensure free of contagious diseases; card given to signify clean bill of health; unfit immigrants may be sent home

**1910** Harrison demonstrates nerve-fibre outgrowth extravitality • Flexner produces poliomyelitis experimentally.• Ricketts shows woodtick is vector of Rocky Mountain Spotted Fever, which he differentiates from typhus • X-ray machine guides a surgeon to remove a nail from a boy's lung

**1911** 1st ante-natal clinic, Boston • Peyton Rous transmits a malignant tumour, as a filterable virus • Cushing describes dyspituitarism

**1912** Children's Bureau established, Washington, DC • Public Health Services • Cushing describes pituitary body & disorders

**1913** Supreme Court denies 'rights' of individuals if inimical to public welfare • American College of Surgeons

**1915** Fitzgerald introduces 'zone therapy' to alleviate certain symptoms & induce numbness

**1917-18** American Commission investigates trench fever

**1922** McCollum & others identify Vitamin D

**1928** Iron lung used for the 1st time in the USA

**1932** Development of 1st vaccine against Yellow Fever

**1933** Anti-beriberi vitamin identified by R Williams & colleagues; produced synthetically in **1936**

**1934** Mixter &. Barr demonstrate role of intervertebral disc herniation in sciatica

**1938** New York is 1st state to pass law requiring medical tests for marriage licences

**1943** Waksman discovers streptomycin, 1st antibiotic effective against TB

**1944** 1st eye bank, New York • 1st successful heart operation on a newborn baby • Waksman discovers antibiotic, streptomycin

**1945** World's 1st fluoridated water supply, Michigan • Vaccine against virus A & B influenza used on US army • Benadryl developed to treat common allergies

**1946** Dr Spock's book *Baby & Child Care*

**1947** Gerty Cori: 1st woman wins Nobel Prize in medicine

**1949** Gross does resection of waretation of aorta

**1950** Green grows skin for grafting from a newborn baby • 1st human kidney transplant by R H Lawler • Murray & colleagues transplant 1st kidneys from deceased to living patients

**1952** Artificial heart 1st used in an operation at Pennsylvania Hospital • Operations & hormone treatment changes a man's sex

**1953** Virologist Dr Salk successfully tests a polio vaccine

**1955** Pincus & others invent contraceptive pill

**1956** 1st successful kidney transplant between identical twins by Merrill & others

**1960** Enders & others develop attennated measles virus vaccine

**1966** Artificial blood invented by Clark & Gollan

**1972** Syphilis Scandal in Alabama

**1976** 1st artificial functioning gene

**1981** AIDS recognised in New York & Los Angeles

**1982** 1st operation to implant artificial heart

**1984** AIDS virus discovered

**1987** Prozac licensed

**1992** Baboon liver transplant

**1995** Cancer supergun may help body's immune system fight tumours

**1997** 1st surviving septuplets born

**1998** Viagra, anti-impotence treatment, approved • 1st surviving octuplets born

**1999** New skin patch test for diabetes • Leech neurones used in a 'living' computer • cloning of 1st human embryo

# BIBLIOGRAPHY

**AND FURTHER READING**

*100 Greatest Medical Discoveries*
Grolier Educational Corp., 1997

ABRAM, RUTH
*Send Us a Lady Physician: Women Doctors in America, 1835-1920*
W.W. Norton & Co, 1985

ACHTERBERG, JEANNE
*Woman as Healer*
Shambhala Publications, 1991

ACKERKNECHT, ERWIN HEINZ
*A Short History of Medicine*
Johns Hopkins University Press, 1982

ACKERMAN, EVELYN BERNETTE
*Health Care in the Parisian Countryside, 1800-1914*
Rutgers University Press, 1990

ADAMS, ANNMARIE
*Architecture in the Family Way: Doctors, Houses and Women, 1870-1900*
McGill Queens University Press, 1996

AIDAN, FRANCIS;
CARDINAL, GASQUET
*The Black Death of 1348 and 1349*
AMS Press, 1977

ALPHEN, J. VAN (EDITOR); ET AL
*Oriental Medicine: An Illustrated Guide to the Asian Arts of Healing*
Shambhala Pubns., 1997

ALTON, GEOFF
*Contemporary Accounts of the Great Plague of London*
Tressell Publications, 1985

AMERICAN MEDICAL ASSOCIATION
*Caring for the Country: A History and Celebration of the First 150 Years of the American Medical Association*
Random House, 1997

ANDRESKI, STANISLAV
*Syphilis, Puritanism and Witch Hunts: Historical Explanations in the Light of Medicine and Psychoanalysis with a Forecast about AIDS*
St Martins Press, 1990

ARMSTRONG, DAVID AND
ELIZABETH METZGER ARMSTRONG
*The Great American Medicine Show*
Prentice Hall, 1991

BAAS, J.H.
*History of Medicine*
R. E. Krieger Pub. Co., 1971

BALY, MONICA E.
*Florence Nightingale and the Nursing Legacy, 2nd edition: Building the Foundations of Modern Nursing and Midwifery*
Bain Bridge Books, 1998

BEINFIELD, HARRIET;
KORNGOLD, EFREM
*Between Heaven and Earth: A Guide to Chinese Medicine*
Ballantine Books, 1992

BELL, E.M.
*Storming the Citadel: The Rise of the Woman Doctor*
Constable & Co., 1953

BENDINER, JESSICA;
BENDINER, ELMER (CONTRIBUTOR)
*Biographical Dictionary of Medicine*
Facts on File, Inc., 1990

BERGE, ANN L.A.;
FEINGOLD, MORDECHAI (EDITOR)
*French Medical Culture in the Nineteenth Century*
Rodopi BV Editions, 1994

BINNEVELD, J.M.W.;
BINNEVELD, HANS
*From Shell Shock to Combat Stress: A Comparative History of Military Psychiatry*
Amsterdam University Press, 1998

BISHOP, W.J.
*The Early History of Surgery, Oldbourne, 1960*

BLAKE, J.B.
*Education in the History of Medicine*
Hafner Publishing Co., 1968

BLISS, MICHAEL
*The Discovery of Insulin*
McClelland & Stewart, 1996

BLUSTEIN, BONNIE ELLEN
*Preserve Your Love for Science* (Life of William Hammond, American Neurologist)
Cambridge University Press, 1992

BONDESON, JAN (PREFACE)
*A Cabinet of Medical Curiosities*
Cornell University Press, 1999

BOURDILLON, HILARY
*Women as Healers: A History of Women and Medicine*
Cambridge University Press, 1989

BOUSELL, PATRICE; BONNEMAIN,
HENRI; BOVÉ, FRANK
*History of Pharmacy and the Pharmaceutical Industry*
Asklepios Press, 1982

BRITISH MEDICAL ASSOCIATION
*Complementary Medicine: New approaches to Good Practice*
BMA, 1993

BROCKINGTON, C.F.
*The Theory and Practice of Public Health*
Oxford University Press, 1975

BROOKE, ELISABETH
*Medicine Women: A Pictorial History of Women Healers*
Quest Books, 1997

BROOKE, ELISABETH
*Women Healers: Portraits of Herbalists, Physicians, and Midwives*
Inner Traditions Int Ltd 1995

BRYAN, JENNY
*The History of Health and Medicine (Science Discovery)*
Thomson Learning, 1996

BRYDER, LINDA
*Below the Magic Mountain: A Social History of Tuberculosis in Twentieth-Century Britain*
(Oxford Historical Monographs)
Oxford University Press, 1988

BULLOUGH, V.L.
*The Development of Medicine as a Profession*
S.Karger, 1966

BUSVINE, JAMES R.
*Disease Transmission by Insects: Its discovery and 90 years of effort to prevent it*
Spring Verlag, 1993

BYNUM, W.F. (EDITOR);
PORTER, ROY (EDITOR)
*Companion Encyclopedia of the History of Medicine*
Routledge, 1997

CAMERON, M.L.
*Anglo-Saxon Medicine* (Cambridge Studies in Anglo-Saxon England, Vol 7),
Cambridge University Press, 1993

CAMPBELL, DONALD
*Arabian Medicine and its Influence on the Middle Ages*
Kegan Paul, Trench, Trüber & Co, 1926

CAMPBELL, SHEILA; ET AL
*Health, Disease and Healing in Medieval Culture*
St Martins Press, 1991

CARTWRIGHT, F.
*The Development of Modern Surgery*
Arthur Baker Ltd 1967

CASSEDY, JAMES H.
*American Medicine and Statistical Thinking, 1800-1860*
Harvard University Press, 1984

CASSEDY, JAMES H.
*Medicine in America: A Short History*
(The American Moment)
Johns Hopkins University Press, 1991

CLIFFORD, THOMAS;
ALLBUTT, SIR
*The Historical Relations of Medicine and Surgery to the End of the 16th Century*
AMS Press, 1978

COCHRANE, JENNIFER
*An Illustrated History of Medicine*
Tiger Books International, 1996

COD, F.E.G.
*Illustrated History of Tropical Diseases*
Wellcome Trust, 1996

COHEN, MARK NATHAN
*Health and the Rise of Civilization*
Yale University Press, 1991

COLEMAN, VERNON
*The Story of Medicine*
Robert Hale, 1985

CONRAD, LI; ET AL
*The Western Medical Tradition 800BC to AD1800*
Cambridge University Press, 1995

COWARD, R.
*The Whole Truth: The Myth of Alternative Medicine*
Faber & Faber, 1989

CRAVENS, HAMILTON (EDITOR)
*Technical Knowledge in American Culture: Science, Technology, and Medicine Since the Early 1800s )*
University of Alabama Press, 1996

CRELLIN, J.K.; PHILPOTT, J,
*Herbal Medicine of Past and Present*
Duke University Press

CRISSEY, JOHN T.
*Dermatology and Syphilology of the Nineteenth Century*
Praeger Pub Text, 1981

CULE, JOHN
*A Doctor for the People: 2000 Years of General Practice in Britain*
Update Books, 1980

CULE, JOHN
*Wales and Medicine: A source list for printed books and papers showing the history of medicine in relation to Wales and Welshmen*
National Library of Wales, 1980

CUMSTON, C.G.
*History of Medicine - The History of Civilization*
Routledge, 1997

d'ESTAING, VALÉRIE-ANNE GISCARD
*The Book of Inventions and Discoveries*
Macdonald Queen Anne Press, 1991

DIGBY, ANNE
*The Evolution of British General Practice 1850-1948*
Oxford University Press, 1999

DUFFY, JOHN
*From Humors to Medical Science: A History of American Medicine*
University of Illinois Press, 1993

DUIN, NANCY; SUTCLIFFE, JENNY
*A History of Medicine*
Simon & Schuster, 1992

DUKE, MARTIN
*The Development of Medical Techniques and Treatments: From Leeches to Heart surgery*
International Universities Press, 1991

DUNLOP, ROBERT H.;
WILLIAMS, DAVID J.,
(CONTRIBUTOR)
*Veterinary Medicine: An Illustrated History*
Mosby Year Book, 1995

EAGLE, R.
*A Guide to Alternative Medicine*
British Broadcasting Corporation, 1980

Eberson, Frederick
*Early Physicians of the West*
Valkyrie Pub. House, 1979

EDELSTEIN, LUDWIG; ET AL
*Ancient Medicine: Selected Papers of Ludwig Edelstein*
Johns Hopkins University Press, 1989

EDWARDS, OWEN DUDLEYS
*Burkes and Hare*
Laurier Books Ltd, 1994

EHRENREICH, BARBARA; ENGLISH,
DEIRDRE
*Witches, Midwives, and Nurses: A History of Women Healers*
Feminist Press, 1973

ELIZABETH FEE (EDITOR); DANIEL
M. FOX (EDITOR)
*AIDS: The Making of a Chronic Disease*
University California Press, 1992

ELLIS, H.
*Operations That Made History*
Greenwich Medical Publications, 1996

ELLIS, H.
*Surgical Case Histories from the Past*
Royal Society of Medicine Press, 1994

EMMERSON, JOAN S. (EDITOR)
*Catalogue of the Pybus Collection of Medical Books, Letters and Engravings: 15th - 20th Centuries*
Manchester University Press, 1983

*Encylcopaedia Britannica*

FELDBERG, GEROGINA D.
*Disease and Class: Tuberculosis and the Shaping of Modern North American Society (Health and Medicine in American Society)*
Rutgers University Press, 1995

FINNANE, MARK
*Insanity and the Insane in Post-Famine Ireland*
Barnes & Noble, 1981

FREEMON, FRANK, R
*Gangrene and Glory: Medical Care During the American Civil War*
Fairleigh Dickinson University Press, 1998

FRENCH, ROGER (EDITOR); ET AL
*Medicine from the Black Death to the French Disease (History of Medicine in Context)*
Ashgate Publishing Co., 1998

FRENCH, ROGER;
WEAR, ANDREW (EDITOR)
*British Medicine in an Age of Reform (Wellcome Institute Series in the History of Medicine)*
Routledge, 1992

FRIEDMAN, MEYER;
FRIEDMAN, GERALD W.
*Medicine's 10 Greatest Discoveries*
Yale University Press, 1998

FURST, LILIAN R. (EDITOR)
*Women Healers and Physicians: Climbing a Long Hill*
University Press of Kentucky, 1997

GABRIEL, RICHARD A.;
METZ, KAREN S.
*A History of Military Medicine*
Greenwood Publishing Group, 1992

GARZA, HEDDA; GREEN, ROBERT
*Women in Medicine (Women Then-Women Now)*
Franklin Watts, Inc, 1996

GENTILCORE, DAVID
*Healers and Healing in Early Modern Italy (Social and Cultural Values in Early Modern Europe)*
Manchester University Press, 1998

GETZ, FAYE MARIE
*Healing and Society in Medieval England: A Middle English Translation of the Pharmaceutical Writings of Gilbertus Anglicus*
University of Wisconsin Press, 1991

GETZ, FAYE
*Medicine in the English Middle Ages*
Princeton University Press, 1998

GIBLIN, JAMES CROSS;
FRAMPTON, DAVID (ILLUSTRATOR)
*When Plague Strikes: The Black Death, Smallpox, AIDS*
Harper Collins Children's Books, 1997

GILMAN, SANDER L.
*Sexuality: An Illustrated History: Representing the Sexual in Medicine and Culture from the Middle Ages to the Age of AIDS*
John Wiley & Sons, 1989

GOLDIE, SUE M. (EDITOR)
*Nightingale, Florence, 'I Have Done My Duty': Florence Nightingale in the Crimean War, 1854-58*
University of Iowa, 1988

GORDON L.
*A Country Herbal*
Mayflower Books, 1980

GORDON, RICHARD
*An Alarming History of Famous and Difficult Patients: Amusing Medical Anecdotes from Typhoid Mary to FDR*
St Martins Press, 1997

GORDON, RICHARD
*The Alarming History of Medicine/Amusing Anecdotes from Hippocrates to Heart Transplants*
St Martins Press, 1994

GREENE, REBECCA (EDITOR)
*History of Medicine*
Hamworth FR, 1988

GRMEK, MIRKO DRAZEN
(EDITOR); ET AL
*Western Medical Thought from Antiquity to the Middle Ages*
Harvard University Press, 1999

GUTHRIE, DOUGLAS
*A History of Medicine*
J.B. Lippincott Co., 1946

HAMILTON, DAVID (INTRODUCTION)
*The Healers: A History of Medicine in Scotland (The Little Books Series)*
Pelican Pub. Co., 1999

HAMLIN, CHRISTOPHER
*Public Health in the Age of Chadwick (Britain 1800-1854)*
Cambridge University Press, 1998

HANAWAY, JOSEPH;
CRUESS, RICHARD (CONTRIBUTOR)
*McGill Medicine: The First Half Century 1829-1885*
McGill Queens University Press, 1996

HANLON, J.J.
*Public Health: Administration and Practice*
C.V. Mosby Co, 1974

HICKS, A.
*Principles of Chinese Medicine*
Thorson, 1996

HO, P.Y.; LISOWSKI, F.P.
*A Brief History of Chinese Medicine and Its Influence*
World Scientific Pub. Co., 1996

HOOPER, TONY.
*Breakthrough Surgery*
Simon & Schuster Young Books, 1992

HORACIO, J.R. FABREGA
*Evolution of Sickness and Healing*
University California Press, 1997

HORROX, ROSEMARY
(TRANSLATOR)
*The Black Death (Manchester Medieval Sources)*
Manchester University Press, 1994

HOWSON, MARK; ET AL
*Practice and How It Fits With the Medicine of the West*
Henry Holt, 1990

HUDSON, ROBERT P.
*Disease and Its Control, The Shaping of Modern Thought*
Greenwood Press, 1983

HUNT, T.
*The Medieval Surgery*
The Boydell Press, 1992

HUNTER, LYNETTE (EDITOR);
HUTTON, SARAH (EDITOR)
*Women, Science and Medicine 1500-1700: Mothers and Sisters of the Royal Society*
Sutton Publishing, 1997

HURD-MEAD, KATE CAMPBELL
*A History of Women in Medicine from the Earliest Times to the Beginning of the Nineteenth Century*
AMS Press, 1977

Hurd-Mead, K.C.
*A History of Women in Medicine*
Milford House, 1973

ISAACS, RONALD H., JUDAISM
*Medicine and Healing*
Cason Aronson, 1998

JACKSON, RALPH
*Doctors and Diseases in the Roman Empire*
University of Oklahoma Press, 1988

JOHNSON, R.W.
*Disease and Medicine*
B.T. Batsford, 1967

JONES, HELEN
*Health and Society in Twentieth-Century Britain (Themes in British Social History)*
Longman Group UK, 1994

Jones, Peter Murray
*Medieval Medicine in Illuminated Manuscripts*
British Library Publications, 1999

JORDANOVA, LUDMILLA
*Sexual Visions: Images of Gender in Science and Medicine Between the Eighteenth and Twentieth Centuries)*
University of Wisconsin Press, 1993

JOUANNA, JACQUES; ET AL
*Hippocrates (Medicine and Culture)*
Johns Hopkins University Press, 1999

KAPTCHUK, T; CROUCHER M.
*The Healing Arts: A journey through the Faces of Medicine*
BBC, 1986

KAUFMAN, SHARON R.
*The Healer's Tale: Transforming Medicine and Culture*
University of Wisconsin Press, 1995

KETT
*The Formation of the American Medical Profession*
Greenwood Publishing Group, 1980

KING, ROGER
*Making of the Dentiste, 1650-1780*
Ashgate Publishing Ltd, 1998

KIPLE, KENNETH, F., (EDITOR)
*The Cambridge World History of Human Disease*
Cambridge University Press, 1993

KIPLE, KENNETH
*Plague, Pox & Pestilence*
Weidenfeld & Nicolson, 1997

KNAPP, VINCENT J.
*Disease and Its Impact on Modern European History (Studies in Health and Human Services, Vol 10)*
Edwin Mellen Press, 1989

KREMERS, E.; URDANG, G.
*History of Pharmacy*
J.B.Lippincott Co., 1976

LAWRENCE, CHRISTOPHER
*Medical Theory, Surgical Practice*
Routledge, 1992

LEATHARD, AUDREY
*Health Care Provision: Past, Present, and Future*
Chapman & Hall, 1990

LEAVITT, JUDITH WALZER
*Typhoid Mary: Captive to the Public's Health*
Beacon Press, 1997

LIPP, MARTIN, R.
*Medical Landmarks USA: A Travel Guide to Historic Sites, Architectural Gems, Remarkable Museums and Libraries, and Other Places Health-Related*
McGraw-Hill, 1990

LISOWSKI, F.P.; Ho, P.Y.
*Brief History of Chinese Medicine, 1997*

LLOYD, WYNDHAM E.B.
*A Hundred Years of Medicine*
Gerald Duckworth & Co Ltd, 1968

LONGRIGG, JAMES (EDITOR)
*Greek Medicine: From the Heroic to the Hellenistic Age: A Source Book*
Routledge, 1998

LOUDON, IRVINE (EDITOR)
*Western Medicine:*
*An Illustrated History*
Oxford University Press, 1997

LOUDON, IRVINE (EDITOR); ET AL
*General Practice Under*
*the National Health Service*
*1948-1997*
Clarendon Press, 1998

LU, HENRY C.
*Chinese System of Natural*
*Cures*
Sterling Publications, 1994

LUCHETTI, CATHY
*Medicine Women:*
*The Story of Early-*
*American Women Doctors*
Crown Publications, 1998

LYONS, A. S;PETRUCELLI, R. J.
*Medicine*
*An Illustrated History*
Abradale Press, Harry N.
Abramd, Inc., Publishers, 1987

MAGNER, LOIS N.
*A History of Medicine*
Marcel Dekker, 1992

MAJOR, RALPH, H.
*A History of Medicine*
Blackwell, 1954

MARCUSE, PETER M.
*Disease:*
*In Search of Remedy*
University of Illinois Press,
1996

MARGOTTA, ROBERTO
*The Hamlyn History*
*of Medicine*
Reed International, 1996

MAYER, ROBERT G.
*Embalming:*
*History, Theory, & Practice*
Appleton & Lange, 1996

MCGOWEN, TOM
*The Black Death*
(First Books)
Franklin Watts, Incorp., 1995

MCGREGOR, DEBORAH KUHN
*From Midwives to Medicine:*
*The Birth of American*
*Gynecology*
Rutgers University Press,
1998

METTLER, CECELIA
*History of Medicine*
Blakiston Co., 1947

MEYER, CLARENCE
*American Folk Medicine*
Meyer Books, 1985

MICHELL, A.R. (EDITOR)
*The Advancement*
*of Veterinary Science:*
*History of the Healing*
*Professions: Parallels*
*Between Veterinary and*
*Medical History*
Cabi Publishing, 1993

MILLER, JONATHAN
*The Body in Question*
Jonathan Cape, 1978

MILLER, TIMOTHY S.
*The Birth of the Hospital*
*in the Byzantine Empire*
Johns Hopkins University
Press, 1997

MORTON, L. T.;MOORE, R. J.
*A Chronology of Medicine*
*and Related Sciences*
Scolar Press, 1997

MOSCUCCI, ORNELLA
*The Science of Woman:*
*Gynaecology and Gender*
*in England, 1800-1929*
Cambridge University Press,
1993

NEWMAN, ART
*The Illustrated Treasury*
*of Medical Curiosa*
McGraw Hill, 1988

NULAND, SHERWIN B
*Medicine The Art of Healing*
Hugh Lauter Levin Associates
Inc., 1992

NUMBERS, RONALD L., (EDITOR);
AMUNDSEN, DARREL W. (EDITOR)
*Caring and Curing: Health*
*and Medicine in the Western*
*Religious Traditions*
Johns Hopkins University
Press, 1998

NUNN, JOHN F.
*Ancient Egyptian Medicine*
University of Oklahoma
Press, 1996

NUTTON, V.; PORTER, ROY
*Murders and Miracles: Lay*
*Attitudes Towards Medicine*
*in Classical Antiquity*
Cambridge University Press,
1985

O'BOYLE, CORNELIUS
*The Art of Medicine:*
*Medical Teaching at the*
*University of Paris, 1250-*
*1400*
Brill Academic Publishers,
1998

ORME, N.; WEBSTER, M.
*The English Hospital*
*1070-1570*
Yale University Press, 1995

PHILLIPS, E.D.
*Aspects of Greek Medicine*
The Charles Press,
Publishers, 1987

PICK, CHRISTOPHER;
MURPHY, DERVLA
*Embassy to Constantinople*
*The Travels of Lady Mary*
*Worley Montagu*
Century, 1988

PICKSTONE, JOHN V (EDITOR)
*Medical Innovations in*
*Historical Perspective*
St Martins Press, 1992

PORTER, DOROTHY
*Health, Civilization and the*
*State: A History of Public*
*Health from Ancient to*
*Modern Times*
Routledge, 1999

PORTER, DOROTHY;
PORTER, ROY (EDITOR)
*Doctors, Politics and*
*Society: Historical Essays*
Rodopi BV Editions, 1993

PORTER, DOROTHY;
PORTER, ROY
*Patient's Progress*
Polity Press (Blackwell
Publishing), 1989

PORTER, ROY (EDITOR)
*Medicine: A History of*
*Healing:*
*Ancient Traditions to*
*Modern Practices*
Michael O'Mara Books, 1997

PORTER, ROY (EDITOR)
*The Cambridge Illustrated*
*History of Medicine*
Cambridge University Press,
1996

PORTER, ROY
*Disease, Medicine and*
*Society in England,*
*1550-1860*
Cambridge University Press,
1996

PORTER, ROY
*Doctor of Society Thomas*
*Beddoes and the Sick*
*Trade in Late*
*Enlightenment England*
Routledge, 1992

PORTER, ROY
*Health for Sale:*
*Quackery in England*
*1660-1850*
Manchester University Press,
1989

PORTER, ROY
*London: A Social History*
Harvard University Press,
1998

PORTER, ROY
*Mind Forg'd Manacles:*
*Madness in England*
*from Restoration to*
*the Regency*
Harvard University Press,
1988

PORTER, ROY
*The Cambridge Illustrated*
*History of Medicine*
Cambridge University Press,
1996

PORTER, ROY
*The Greatest Benefit to*
*Mankind:*
*A Medical History of*
*Humanity*
W.W. Norton & Co.
1998

PORTER, ROY; PORTER, DOROTHY
*In Sickness and in Health:*
*The British Experience,*
*1650-1850*
Blackwell Pub., 1989

POUCHELLE, MARIE-CHRISTINE
*The Body and Surgery in*
*the Middle Ages*
Rugers University Press,
1990

POWELL, J.H.; ET AL
*Bring Out Your Dead:*
*The Great Plague of Yellow*
*Fever in Philadelphia*
*in 1793*
University of Pennsylvania
Press, 1993

Poynter, F.N.L.
*Medicine and Culture*
Wellcome Institute for the
History of Medicine, 1969

PREUSS, JULIUS;
ROSNER, FRED (TRANSLATOR)
*Biblical and Talmudic*
*Medicine*
Jason Aronson, 1994

PRIORESCHI, PLINIO
*A History of Medicine:*
*Greek Medicine*
*(Mellen History of Medicine)*
Edwin Mellen Press, 1994

PRIORESCHI, PLINIO
*The History of Medicine:*
*Primitive and Ancient*
*Medicine*
(Mellen History of Medicine,
Vol.1)
Edwin Mellen Press, 1991

PROCTOR, ROBERT N
*The Nazi War on Cancer*
Princeton University Press,
1999

RAWCLIFFE, CAROLE
*Medicine & Society in Later*
*Medieval England*
Sutton Publishing, 1998

*Readers' Digest Family Guide*
*to Alternative Medicine*
The Reader's Digest
Association Ltd, 1991

REAGAN, LESLIE J.
*When Abortion Was a Crime:*
*Women, Medicine, and Law in*
*the United States, 1867-1973*
University of California Press,
1998

REPP, PROFESSOR REPP
*Timelines of World History*
Bramley Books, 1998

Reynolds, Brenda, M.
*History of Medicine: Reference*
*and Research Subject*
*Analysis With Bibliography*
ABBE Publishers Association
of Washington DC, 1984

REYNOLDS, MOIRA DAVISON
*How Pasteur Changed*
*History: The Story of Louis*
*Pasteur and the Pasteur*
*Institute*
McGuinn & McGuire
1994

RHODES, PHILIP
*An Outline History*
*of Medicine*
Butterworth, 1985

RIDDLE, J.M.
*Dioscordies on Pharmacy*
*and Medicine*
University of Texas Press,
1985

RILEY, JAMES C.
*The Eighteenth Century*
*Campaign to Avoid Disease*
St Martins Press, 1987

ROBERTS, CHARLOTTE;
MANCHESTER, KEITH
(CONTRIBUTOR)
*The Archaeology of Disease*
Cornell University Press,
1997

ROBERTS, SHIRLEY
*Sophia Jex-Blake (A woman*
*Pioneer in Nineteenth Century*
*Medical Reform)*
Routledge, 1993

ROCCATAGLIATA, GUIEPPE, *A*
*History of Ancient*
*Psychiatry*
Greenwood Publishing
Group, 1986

ROOT-BERNSTEIN, ROBERT; ET AL
*Honey, Mud, Maggots, and*
*Other Medical Marvels:*
*The Science Behind Folk*
*Remedies and Old Wives'*
*Tales*
Mariner Books, 1998

ROSE, JEANNE
*A History of Herbs and*
*Herbalism: A Chronology*
*from 10,000 BC to the*
*Present*
Herbal Studies Course, 1988

ROSENBERG, CHARLES E.
*Explaining Epidemics:*
*And Other Studies in the*
*History of Medicine*
Cambridge University Press,
1992

ROSENBERG, C E.; GOLDEN, J.
*Framing Disease: Studies in*
*Cultural History (Health and*
*Medicine in American Society)*
Rutgers University Press,
1992

ROSENFELD, LOUIS
*Thomas Hodgkin: Morbid*
*Anatomist & Social Activist*
Madison Books, 1993

ROSNER, LISA
*Medical Education in the*
*Age of Improvement:*
*Edinburgh Students and*
*Apprentices 1760-1826*
Edinburgh University Press,
1991

ROTHSTEIN, WILLIAM G.
*American Physicians in the*
*Nineteenth Century:*
*From Sects to Science*
Johns Hopkins University
Press, 1992

ROUSSELOT, JEAN
*Medicine in Art:*
*A Cultural History*
McGraw-Hill, 1967

RUSHTON, ALAN R.
*Genetics and Medicine in*
*the United States 1800 to*
*1922*
Johns Hopkins University
Press, 1994